The Critically Ill Neurosurgical Patient

CONTEMPORARY ISSUES IN CRITICAL CARE NURSING VOLUME 3

The Critically Ill Neurosurgical Patient

Edited by

Diana L. Nikas, R.N., M.N., C.C.R.N., C.N.R.N.

Assistant Professor
Critical Care Clinical Specialist Program
California State University, Long Beach
Clinical Nurse Specialist, Neurology-Neurosurgery
Los Angeles County—University of Southern
California Medical Center
Los Angeles, California

Churchill Livingstone
NEW YORK, EDINBURGH, LONDON, AND MELBOURNE 1982

Distributed in the United Kingdom by Churchill Livingstone, Robert Stevenson House, 1-3 Baxter's Place, Leith Walk, Edinburgh EH1 3AF and by associated companies, branches and representatives throughout the world.

First published 1982

Printed in USA

ISBN 0-443-08158-1

7   6   5   4   3   2

Library of Congress Cataloging in Publication Data

Main entry under title:

The critically ill neurosurgical patient.

    (Contemporary issues in critical care nursing; v.3)
    Bibliography: p.
    Includes index.
    1. Nervous system—Surgery—Complications and sequelae.
2. Critical care medicine.   I. Nikas, Diana L.   II. Series.
[DNLM: 1. Nervous system diseases—Nursing.
WI CO769MQM v.3 WY 160 C934]
RD593.C68   1982   617′.4801   82-14746
ISBN 0-443-08158-1

Contributors

Mary Blount, R.N., M.N., F.A.A.N.
Assistant Director, Department of Nursing, University of Virginia,
Charlottesville, Virginia

Anna Belle Kinney, R.N., M.N., C.N.R.N.
Clinical Nurse Specialist, Neurosurgery, Department of Nursing, University
of Virginia, Charlottesville, Virginia

Mary Pat Lovely, R.N., M.N., C.N.R.N.
Clinical Nurse Specialist, Neurology, Seattle, Washington

Nancy Luttrell, R.N., M.S., C.C.R.N.
Graduate Student, School of Nursing, University of Virginia,
Charlottesville, Virginia

Ellen McCarthy, R.N., M.S., C.C.R.N.
Assistant Professor, Critical Care Clinical Nurse Specialist Program,
California State University, Long Beach, California

Pamela H. Mitchell, M.S., C.N.R.N., F.A.A.N.
Professor, Department of Physiological Nursing, Neurological Nurse
Specialist, Division of Neurology, Research Affiliate, Regional Primate
Center, University of Washington, Seattle, Washington

Diana L. Nikas, R.N., M.N., C.C.R.N., C.N.R.N.
Assistant Professor, Critical Care Clinical Specialist Program, California
State University, Long Beach, Clinical Nurse Specialist,
Neurology–Neurosurgery, Los Angeles County–University of Southern
California Medical Center, Los Angeles, California

Judy Ozuna, R.N., M.N., C.N.R.N.
Clinical Nurse Specialist, and Supervisor, Epilepsy, Harborview Medical
Center, Clinical Nurse Specialist, Neurology, Veterans Administration
Medical Center, Seattle, Washington

Marilyn M. Ricci, R.N., B.S., C.N.R.N.
Clinical Nurse Specialist, Neurology–Neurosurgery, Barrow Neurological
Institute, Phoenix, Arizona

Sarah J. Sanford, R.N., M.A., C.C.R.N.
Associate Director Nursing (Medical, Surgical, Critical Care) Overlake
Memorial Hospital, Bellevue, Washington

Carol Salminen, R.N., B.S.N.
Nurse Epidemiologist, Neurosurgical Service, Los Angeles
County–University of Southern California Medical Center, Los Angeles,
California

Mary Tolley, R.N., A.A.
Head Nurse, Medical Clinics, Los Angeles County–University of Southern
California Medical Center, Los Angeles, California

Nancy Wanski, R.N., M.N., C.C.R.N.
Critical Care Clinical Nurse Specialist, Los Angeles, California

Contents

The Critically Ill Neurosurgical Patient

1 | Neurological Examination and Assessment of Altered States of Consciousness

Marilyn M. Ricci

The integrity of the nervous system may be altered by a wide variety of pathological entities. Anatomical and/or physiological disruption may result from primary disease of the nervous system or as a complication of systemic disease. Involvement of the structures that support, protect, and nourish the nervous system may precipitate neurologic dysfunction or compromise neurologic integrity.

The nervous system receives sensory stimuli from the environment, transmits motor responses, maintains communication between body parts, interprets at reflex and conscious levels, and integrates all body activities. The clinical picture associated with neurologic impairment is a combination of intact functions and the inability to receive, interpret, transmit and/or integrate information appropriately.

A neurological evaluation is performed to determine the presence or absence of dysfunction, the location and etiology of the pathological process, the status of the neurological deficits, the potential threat to survival, the highest degree of functional ability, and the influence of the disability on the patient's

1

life-style. A comprehensive approach to the neurological evaluation comprises a detailed patient history and a systematic neurologic examination that includes evaluation of mentation, language, motor, sensory, reflex, and autonomic activities.

HISTORY

A complete patient and family history will provide valuable clues which will enable more effective clinical examination, problem analysis, and patient management. The patient should be the primary source of the historical data. The family members/friends should be utilized to obtain information particularly in the presence of language disturbance, defective memory, depressed conscious level, or other cognitive deficits. Significant historical data include any familial/hereditary disease, previous trauma, and cardiovascular, infectious, or metabolic disease.

Identification of the major symptoms, their onset, progression, and chronology will assist in determining the etiology and management. Symptoms may increase in severity or variety, may plateau or subside, depending on the nature of the disease process. Symptoms gain significance as they appear in combination with other specific symptoms, and in conjunction with the information obtained from the neurological examination. An abrupt onset of symptoms is characteristic of head injury, meningitis, viral encephalitis, and cerebral hemorrhage or embolization. Rapid progression is commonly seen with malignant brain tumors and viral encephalitis. Sporadic remission, periods of stability, and recurrence of symptoms are characteristic of ischemic-occlusive disease and some degenerative states.[1]

Headache and pain are frequent presenting symptoms of neurological disorders. The location may be focal, unilateral, bilateral, or generalized. The description may vary markedly from patient to patient. Transient headache may precede cerebral hemorrhage, but a "blinding, bursting" headache of sudden onset can herald a subarachnoid hemorrhage. An early morning headache often occurs with brain tumors. A patient who complains of headache and also has a fever is suggestive of meningitis, encephalitis, or systemic disease; without fever, headache suggests an aneurysm, subarachnoid hemorrhage, or an intracranial tumor.[1]

Other common neurologically induced symptoms requiring evaluation include visual loss, diplopia, dizziness, vertigo, numbness, weakness, defective memory, language impairment, and depressed conscious level.

MENTATION

Mentation consists of conscious level or arousability and cognition. These activities reflect generalized brain integrity. Conscious level is represented by the individual's ability to maintain contact with the environment and respond to environmental stimuli, and the quality of verbalizations. The general appearance, facial expression, manner of speech, mood, affect, and general behavior provide clues to the patient's mentation. Components of the cognitive level include attention span; orientation to time, place, and person; immediate recall and memory for recent and remote events; ability to understand; intellectual performance; judgment, perception, and general knowledge.

Mentation is evaluated during the initial patient contact. Responsiveness to verbal stimuli permits an in-depth evaluation of the cognitive status. Decreased responsiveness limits the cognitive evaluation and requires a more extensive evaluation of the conscious level (see section on Altered States of Consciousness). Cognitive status is evaluated by asking the patient for specific information about himself or herself, past historical events, and details from the previous few minutes. Provide an opportunity to repeat digits, problem-solve, interpret proverbs, and discuss well-known events or people. These techniques will demonstrate the functional integrity of the frontal and temporal lobes. Consideration must be given to previous educational background and experience of the patient.

The clinical indications of frontal lobe involvement are withdrawal from and disinterest in the environment, impaired judgment, loss of insight, decreased reasoning ability, confusion, labile emotional responses, and loss of vast amounts of information about people, events, and past experiences. Temporal lobe dysfunction usually alters the ability to return information, and affects recent memory, the ability to learn, and personality. The degree to which conscious level and cognition is altered is directly related to the extent of loss of functional integrity of the cerebral hemispheres and brainstem.

LANGUAGE

Language is a highly complex mode of communication that enables the individual to acquire and transmit information. Verbal, written, and numerical symbols and gestures are used to express thoughts. The symbols must be recognized, interpreted, and responses should be initiated to execute the communication process. Recognition and usage of common objects are included as language skills. Multiple areas of the brain participate in the integrated function of language, however, the left cerebral hemisphere is the primary language center in most people. The right hemisphere plays a major role in visual/spatial perception, the appreciation of nonverbal information, and processing of information.[2]

An evaluation of language skills begins with the initial patient contact, and requires an alert responsive patient. The ability for spontaneous speech, word usage, and fluency is evaluated; the ability to repeat words, phrases, and sentences is evaluated; the ability to follow serial commands, read with understanding, write, recognize, name, and use common objects (e.g., pen, pencil, key, and coins) is tested. Interpretation of the language evaluation must be done in view of the sensory and motor deficits since impaired vision, hearing, proprioception, muscle strength, and coordination all influence language.

Lesions in the left temporoparietal area (Wernicke's area) will result in impaired comprehension of the spoken and written word (sensory dysphasia). Lesions of the left frontal area (Broca's area) are characterized by the inability to verbalize formulated thoughts, even though the musculature of articulation and phonation are intact (motor dysphasia). Paresis/paralysis of the laryngeal, pharyngeal, and tongue musculature are characterized by slurred speech and loss of tonal quality (dysarthria). Jerky, irregular speech is consistent with cerebellar pathology.

Visual recognition of the symbols used in reading, writing, and calculation originates in the left parietal lobe. Loss of function in this area is characterized by impaired reading ability (dyslexia), impaired writing ability (dysgraphia), and inability to calculate (acalcula). Lesions of the angular gyrus of the parietal lobe will result in the inability to recognize and interpret sensory stimuli (agnosia) and may be visual, auditory, and/or tactile in nature, depending on which association pathways are involved. The ability to execute planned motor acts is a parietal lobe function. Lesions in this area produce the inability to program volitional activities (apraxia) which include speech, writing, drawing, and assembling.[2]

The overall approach to language evaluation should include a determination of the patient's existing ability to understand and to express himself or herself. The degree and extent of the deficits will vary considerably from patient to patient. Use the existing ability to establish an effective communication system between the patient and his environment.

CRANIAL NERVES

The cranial nerves have sensory, motor, and reflex functions. Each pair of cranial nerves should be examined individually and consecutively because of their complexities.

Olfactory Nerve—I

The function of the olfactory nerve is smell. Test each nostril separately by having the patient sniff aromatic, volatile, nonirritating substances such as coffee, lemon, and peppermint. Avoid the use of ammonia.

Loss of smell (anosmia) occurs with frontal lobe lesions, anterior fossa trauma, or surgery, e.g., pituitary tumor. Indications of anosmia may include complaints of an inability to taste food and/or disinterest in eating.[3]

Optic Nerve—II

Optic nerve functions include visual acuity, peripheral vision, and forms the afferent limb of the pupillary and blink or menace reflexes. Visual disturbances may result from involvement of the optic nerves, the optic chiasm, and the fibers of the optic tract, which transmit visual impulses posteriorly to the occipital cortex. The type and extent of the visual loss will depend on the location of the lesion within the visual pathways.

Visual Acuity. To test distant vision, have the patient read the Snellen Chart at 20 feet. Near vision is tested by having the patient read test cards or newspaper print, or count fingers. Blindness or blurred vision may indicate involvement of the retina, optic disc, optic nerve, optic chiasm, or occipital cortex. Edema of the optic disc (papilledema), which is caused by optic nerve tumors, venous obstruction, and increased intracranial pressure, results in minimal to no loss of visual acuity.[4]

Visual Fields. Gross testing of visual fields is performed by confrontation. The patient is instructed to cover one eye and fix his or her gaze on the examiner's nose. The examiner brings a finger or other object along the axis of the temporal, nasal, superior, and inferior visual fields. The patient indicates when the object is seen.

Partial loss of the visual field or blindness in half of the visual field in one or both eyes is called hemianopia. When a quarter of the visual field is affected, it is called quadrantanopia. Midline involvement of the optic chiasm will produce loss of the temporal visual fields in both eyes (bitemporal hemianopia). Total involvement of the optic tracts and optic radiations in one hemisphere will produce contralateral visual field loss in both eyes (homonymous hemianopia). Partial involvement of the optic chiasm is characterized by bitemporal quadrantanopia. An upper or lower homonymous quadrantanopia is characteristic of partial involvement of the optic tracts or optic radiations. (Fig. 1-1).

Reflexes. The optic nerve forms the afferent limb of the pupillary and menace reflexes, therefore impaired transmission of visual impulses along the optic nerve and the optic tracts will alter the reflex responses. The examiner will be unable to elicit the direct light pupil reflex in a blind eye (See section on Oculomotor Nerve for pupil reflex testing).

Testing of the menace reflex may be accomplished by approaching the patient's eye unexpectedly from the side. Normally, the eyelids will close immediately unless there is impaired visual impulse transmission and/or the inability to close the eyelids.

Oculomotor Nerve—III, Trochlear Nerve—IV, Abducens Nerve—VI

The functions of the oculomotor nerve include elevation of the upper eyelids, pupillary constriction, and eye movements. The oculomotor nerve works in conjunction with the trochlear and abducens nerves, and has cortical pathways which influence voluntary and reflex eye movements.

Eyelids. Observe the eyelids for symmetry. Drooping of the eyelid (ptosis) occurs in the presence of weakness or paralysis of the superior levator palpebrae muscle. Ipsilateral ptosis is characteristic of compression or trauma to the oculomotor nerve, and contralateral ptosis is associated with damage to the cerebral hemisphere. Bilateral ptosis may be seen in patients with neu-

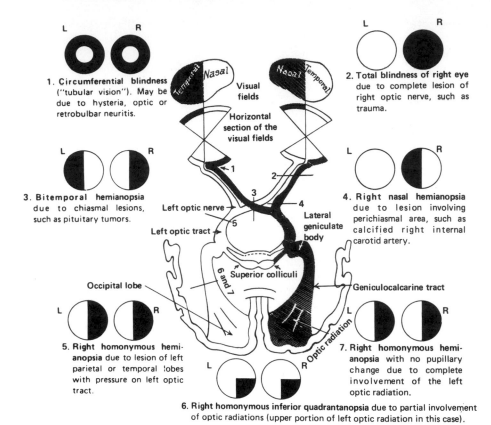

Fig. 1-1. Visual field defects associated with lesions of visual system. (From Chusid JG: Correlative Neuroanatomy & Functional Neurology, 17th ed. Copyright 1979 by Lange Medical Publications, Los Altos, California.)

romuscular disorders such as myasthenia gravis, or Guillain-Barré syndrome, and fatigue.[3]

Pupils. Pupillary functions are dependent on the integrity of the optic pathways, the oculomotor nerves, the brainstem centers, the sympathetic fibers, and the occipital cortical connections. Examination of the pupils includes their size, equality, and reflex activities.

Normal pupil size varies from 1.5 to 6 mm in diameter. The pupil size represents a balance between parasympathetic and sympathetic innervation. Exact measurement of the pupil is the most reliable method of determining size and equality. Unequal pupils (anisocoria) occur from disruption of the parasympathetic fibers of the oculomotor nerve and nucleus (e.g., compression by an aneurysm, tentorial herniation) or from disruption of the sympathetic pathways (e.g., cervical cord trauma). The ipsilateral pupil will be dilated and nonreactive to light with pressure on the parasympathetic pathways of the oculomotor nerve. The ipsilateral pupil will be constricted with an absent ciliospinal reflex due to loss of sympathetic innervation, but will retain the direct light reflex (e.g., Horner's syndrome).

The pupillary reflexes include the direct and consensual light reflexes, the accommodation reflex, and the ciliospinal reflex. The *light reflex* is evaluated by using a bright penlight with dim surrounding lighting, instructing the patient to look straight ahead if possible, and approaching the eye from the side. The pupils should constrict promptly in response to the light. The most important factor is whether or not the pupils react rather than the rate of reaction; however, in early involvement of the oculomotor nerve, the pupil response may be slowed. When determining the *direct light* reflex, each eye must be examined independently with the opposite eye covered. In the event of a swollen eyelid or ptosis, the eyelid may be gently retracted to elicit the light reflex. Loss of light transmission via the optic nerve results in loss of the direct light reflex, although the consensual reflex will be intact. Progressive dilatation and loss of the direct light reflex and consensual reflex is usually indicative of an expanding intracranial mass on that side.

The *consensual light* reflex is determined by shining the light into one eye and observing the opposite eye for constriction. The consensual reflex will remain intact as long as the oculomotor parasympathetic fibers and midbrain connections are intact. Loss of light transmission to the retina (cataract) or optic nerve damage will result in blindness in that eye, but the consensual light reflex will be retained. A patient with blindness due to destruction of the occipital cortex will have normal direct and consensual reflexes.

Accommodation or reflex pupil constriction and convergence in response to near vision is tested by asking the patient to look at a distant object and then at a near object. This reflex is lost with involvement of the occipital cortex.

The *ciliospinal reflex* is defined as ipsilateral pupil dilatation in response to the use of noxious stimulation (pinching) of the neck. This reflex is lost when the sympathetic pathways in the cervical spinal cord or cervical sympathetic chain are damaged (e.g., trauma).[3]

Eye Movements.   The ability to move each eye horizontally, vertically, and at 45 degrees in a conjugate manner is dependent on the integrity of the oculomotor, trochlear and abducens nerves, the brainstem structures, the cortical connections to the frontal and occipital lobes and the cerebellum.

Eye movements are tested by instructing the patient to look upward, downward, and to each side, by following the examiner's finger. Disturbances of eye movements include loss of voluntary or reflex conjugate gaze, deviation of the eyes, and nystagmus.

Extraocular muscle weakness or paralysis and loss of conjugate gaze in a conscious patient results in double vision (diplopia). The patient may complain of dizziness or may be observed tilting his head to compensate for the diplopia. Involvement of specific cranial nerves and/or their nuclei may result in a deviation of one or both eyes (strabismus), dysconjugate gaze, and loss of convergence. Paralysis of the extraocular muscles supplied by the oculomotor nerve produces an inability to deviate the eye upward, downward, and inward. Dysfunction of the trochlear nerve results in weakness of downward gaze. Abducens nerve involvement produces an inability to move the eyes laterally. Loss of coordination of the extraocular movements by the nerves and the vestibular apparatus results in the inability to move the eyes across the midline.[4]

Patients with cerebral hemisphere damage may be unable to look toward the side of the lesion or follow a moving object either on command or reflexively. When the eyes are at rest, a destructive lesion of the frontal or occipital lobes produces conjugate deviation toward the lesion. Conjugate deviation away from the side of a hemispheric lesion is characteristic of an epileptogenic focus or brainstem injury.[4]

Nystagmus or rhythmic, involuntary eye movements may occur at rest or be induced by eye movements. They may be horizontal, vertical, or rotary. Nystagmus occurs as a normal response to gazing at objects moving rapidly across the visual field (optokinetic). It may also be congenital, associated with blindness, or the result of vestibular and cerebellar dysfunction. Drugs such as phenytoin sodium (Dilantin®), phenobarbital, and alcohol may induce nystagmus.[5]

Trigeminal Nerve—V

The trigeminal nerve divides into ophthalmic, maxillary, and mandibular branches, and has both sensory and motor functions. Sensory fibers transmit tactile, pain, temperature, and proprioceptive impulses from the face, cornea, nasal and oral mucosa, sinuses, teeth, tongue, external auditory canal, and meninges. The motor fibers in association with cortical connections innervate the masseter and temporal muscles and control opening and closing of the jaw. Examination includes facial sensation, motor strength of the jaw, the corneal reflex, and the jaw jerk reflex.

Sensation.   Sensation is tested with a wisp of cotton or pinprick over both sides of the face and each of the three divisions of the trigeminal nerve while the patient's eyes are closed. Loss of sensation may occur in one or all three divisions or parts of each division (onionskin type distribution), depending on the location of the lesion. Parietal lobe involvement may result in the inability to interpret sensations (loss of discrimination). Pathology along the peripheral course of the nerve is usually characterized by severe pain on one or all divisions, e.g., trigeminal neuralgia.

Motor.   To test motor strength, the patient is asked to open his or her jaw and to bite down tightly. Deviation of the jaw occurs toward the weak side. While the teeth are clenched, palpation of the temporal and masseter muscles should reveal bilateral contractions. The patient can also be asked to move his jaw laterally against pressure to confirm unilateral weakness or paralysis. Impaired ability to bite down or chew will influence the patient's eating ability and nutritional status. Excessive muscle tone, characteristic of a lesion of the cortical pathways (upper motor neuron), will produce tight clenching of the teeth and difficulty with jaw opening.

Corneal Reflex.   The ophthalmic division of the trigeminal nerve forms the afferent limb of the corneal reflex. Stroking the cornea with a wisp of cotton while the patient looks upward should result in prompt bilateral blinking. Decrease or loss of the protection provided by the corneal reflex can result in significant corneal damage.

Jaw Jerk Reflex.   The jaw jerk reflex is tested by tapping the lower jaw with a finger or reflex hammer when it is slightly open and relaxed to elicit jaw closure. The jaw jerk will be increased in patients with loss of cortical control over the trigeminal nerve.

Facial Nerve—VII

The facial nerve innervates the muscles of facial expression, the motor response associated with the blink and corneal reflexes, and the salivary and lacrimal glands; it also transmits the sense of taste from the anterior two-thirds of the tongue.

Motor.   Examination of the facial nerve includes observation of the face for asymmetry of facial expression, sagging of the lower eyelid, and an inability to close the eye completely. The facial nerve is tested by asking the patient to wrinkle his or her forehead, raise eyebrows, wink, keep eyes closed against resistance, blow cheeks out, show teeth, smile, and whistle. Damage to the facial nerve or its nucleus will produce ipsilateral weakness with asymmetrical facial movements involving the entire side. The blink and corneal reflex will also be absent. Damage to the cortical neurons and their projections results in preservation of upper facial activity with loss of function in the lower face on the contralateral side. A patient with ipsilateral or bilateral facial weakness or paralysis is unable to whistle and show his teeth, and may have a speech impairment, drooling, and difficulty handling food. The patient may complain of "scratchy" eyes and dry mouth. The facial nerve is often affected in patients with Guillain-Barré syndrome or myasthenia gravis.

Taste.   Patients with suspicion of facial nerve pathology should be tested for their sense of taste by placing sweet (sugar), sour (vinegar), salty and bitter (quinine) solutions on the tongue.

Acoustic—VIII

The acoustic nerve is composed of a cochlear division and a vestibular division. The functions of the cochlear division include hearing and conduction of sound. The function of the vestibular division is equilibrium.

Hearing.   The ear, the cochlear nerves, and complex brainstem pathways transmit impulses to the temporal cortical areas in the cerebral hemispheres. Hearing acuity may be tested grossly by rubbing the thumb and index finger together, snapping the fingernail, placing a watch or whispering outside each external auditory meatus with the other ear covered. Cortical lesions do not cause deafness unless they are bilateral, however there may be loss of appreciation of specific sounds and noises. Hearing is absent in the presence of severe nerve damage.

Conduction.   Sound is conducted by both air and bone, although air conduction is usually more efficient than bone conduction. Conduction is tested by placing the stem of a vibrating tuning fork on the mastoid bone until the patient reports that the sound has stopped, then place the tuning fork opposite the external auditory meatus (Rinne's test). Normally the sound will continue to be heard via air conduction. Cochlear nerve involvement is characterized by diminution of both air conduction and bone conduction. Bone conduction will be better than air conduction in the presence of an obstruction of the auditory canal or middle ear disease.

For the Weber's test, place a vibrating tuning fork on the middle of the forehead or the vertex of the head and ask the patient to indicate on which side the sound is best heard. Normally the sound appears to originate in the midline. Lateralization of sound to the opposite side is characteristic of lesions involving the cochlear nerve (nerve deafness). Lateralization of sound to the same side occurs with obstruction of the auditory canal or middle ear disease.

Equilibrium.   Equilibrium is controlled by the vestibular division of the acoustic nerve with its brainstem connections, the cerebellum, and the pathways that communicate with other cranial nerves, the upper cervical nerves, and the cerebral cortex.

The illusion of movement (vertigo) and nystagmus frequently accompanies vestibular nerve dysfunction. Vestibular nerve function may be tested by irrigating the external auditory canal with warm or cold water (caloric testing). The normal response is nystagmus away from and deviation of the eyes toward the side irrigated with cold water. Absence of nystagmus and eye deviation plus vertigo confirms vestibular nerve damage on that side. A patient with loss of consciousness may have caloric testing performed to determine the integrity of the brainstem pathways; however, the clinical reaction of the patient will differ from that of a conscious individual.

Glossopharyngeal Nerve—IX and Vagus Nerve—X

The glossopharyngeal nerve transmits the sense of taste from the posterior one-third of the tongue, and forms the afferent limb of the gag and carotid sinus reflexes. The vagus nerve innervates the muscles of the larynx, pharynx, and soft palate. It also contains parasympathetic fibers which are distributed to the thoracic and abdominal viscera, and fibers which transmit sensory visceral information, e.g., abdominal distention, nausea, depth of respirations, and the quality of the blood pressure. The vagus nerve forms the efferent limb of the gag and carotid sinus reflexes. Since the glossopharyngeal nerve functions as the sensory counterpart to the motor fibers of the vagus nerve, they are tested together.

Taste.   The posterior one-third of the tongue may be tested by using the same solutions as for the facial nerve and should be done at the same time.

Pharynx/Larynx.   Vagal impairment may cause a disturbance of phonation (voice quality) and articulation. Laryngeal paralysis produces hoarseness of the voice, loss of the higher tones, and inspiratory stridor. The soft palate and pharynx are inspected and the patient requested to say "ah" to determine if the uvula is in midline and to test the gag reflex. Dysfunction includes unequal palatal elevation with deviation of the uvula to one side. Difficulty swallowing (dysphagia), nasal regurgitation, choking may also result and will potentiate the threat of aspiration. The sensory disturbances associated with vagal impairment include laryngeal and pharyngeal pain, paresthesias, and anesthesia.

Gag Reflex. The gag reflex is tested by stimulating the pharyngeal wall. The normal response is "retching." Excessive stimulation may produce vomiting since the gag reflex is part of the vomiting mechanism. Injury to the nerves will produce loss of the gag reflex and dysphagia, which increases the possibility of aspiration.

Visceral Reflexes. The visceral reflexes, which are under the influence of the glossopharyngeal and vagus nerves, include the carotid sinus reflex and the oculocardiac reflex. Test the carotid sinus reflex by placing pressure over the carotid sinus. To test the oculocardiac reflex, place pressure on the eyeball. The normal response for both reflexes is slowing of the heart and a decrease in blood pressure. Loss of vagal reflex control produces tachycardia, dyspnea, and dilatation of the stomach. Vagal irritation produces bradycardia and coughing.

Spinal Accessory Nerve—XI

The spinal accessory nerve, in conjunction with the motor fibers of the upper five cervical cord segments, innervates the sternocleidomastoid (SCM) and trapezius muscles to enable flexion and turning of the head and elevation of the shoulders, respectively. Fibers also join the vagus nerve to innervate the laryngeal musculature. The SCM and trapezius muscles are evaluated for symmetry of size, contour, strength, and tone. The SCM muscle is tested by asking the patient to turn his head to each side and palpating the opposite muscle. The trapezius muscle is tested by asking the patient to shrug his or her shoulders against resistance. Symmetrical muscle strength and contractions are normally present. A unilateral paralysis is characterized by atrophy, drooping of the shoulder on that side, and weakness in shoulder shrugging, shoulder elevation, and tilting the head to the same side. Spasticity is characteristic of lesions of the cortical pathways.

Hypoglossal—XII

The hypoglossal nerve controls the musculature of the tongue. The patient is requested to stick out his tongue and move it quickly from side to side. The tongue is normally in midline, symmetrical, and moves rhythmically. Test the strength of the tongue muscles by having the patient push the tip of his tongue against the inside of his cheek on each side, against the resistance of the examiner's hand. Unilateral impairment of hypoglossal function may result in deviation from the midline, atrophy, tremors, weakness, and slow, spastic, irregular, uncoordinated movements. The patient's speech pattern may be explosive, thick, dysarthric, or have a typical "hot-potato-in-the-mouth" sound. Bilateral paralysis will also produce difficulty swallowing and chewing food.

When examining the cranial nerves, inspect the tongue and oral mucosa for evidence of scarring or lacerations from seizure activity, drying due to dehydration, "beefy" redness associated with vitamin B deficiencies, and evidence of other underlying systemic disease.

MOTOR EXAMINATION

Motor activities are under the influence of the motor cortex, basal ganglia, and cerebellum and involve both pyramidal and extrapyramidal pathways. Motor function is evaluated by systematically examining muscle bulk, strength or voluntary active movements, tone or resistance to passive movements, coordination, posture, station, gait, and observing for the presence of abnormal motor activities.

Muscle Bulk

Corresponding muscle groups are inspected for symmetry. These include the trunk, intercostals, diaphragm, and abdominal musculature as well as the muscles of the extremities. Less obvious asymmetry of major muscles of the extremities may be identified by measuring and comparing the muscle circumference. Loss of muscle bulk (atrophy) is usually due to peripheral nerve (lower motor neuron) involvement; however, cortical dysfunction may produce disuse atrophy. Patients with cervical cord injury or Guillain-Barré syndrome may have decreased respiratory excursion with weakness or paralysis of intercostal movements. This is characterized by diaphragmatic breathing with the ribs sucking in on inspiration, low diaphragm, and bulging abdominal muscles. Muscle hypertrophy may occur as a compensatory response to weakness of other muscle groups.

Muscle Strength

Muscle strength must be evaluated in view of the "normal" muscle power for that individual. There will be a considerable variation on the basis of age and usual activity. Muscle strength is tested against resistance, against gravity, and with the effects of gravity removed. The patient is asked to perform voluntary activities, e.g., raise both arms, squeeze the examiner's fingers for a few seconds and then release, flex hips, and push with feet against the examiner's hands. Note if the arm, grip, and leg strength are bilaterally equal and whether they are strong or weak (see Table 1-1).

Handedness should be determined, since the grip is usually slightly stronger in the dominant hand. Subtle weakness and inequality of arm strength will be determined if the arm or arms drift downward when the patient holds them with palms up in front of him and with the eyes closed. Attempts to push the patient's outstretched arms down, and flexion and extension of the arms

Table 1-1. Relationship of Spinal Cord Segments to Functional Ability, Specific Muscles, and Peripheral Nerves

Major Spinal Cord Segments	Functional Ability	Specific Muscles	Peripheral Nerves
C3, 4, 5	Diaphragm excursion	Diaphragm	Phrenic nerve
C5	Shoulder shrug	Trapezius	Spinal accessory nerve
C5, 6	Arm elevation	Deltoid	Auxilliary nerve
	Supinated forearm flexion	Bicepsbrachii	Musculocutaneous nerve
	Neutral forearm flexion	Brachioradialis	Radial nerve
C6, 7, 8	Forearm extension	Triceps	Radial nerve
	Wrist extension	Extensor carpi radialis and ulnaris	Radial nerve
C7, 8	Wrist flexion	Flexor carpi radialis and ulnaris	Radial nerve
C8, T1	Grip	Adductor pollicis	Median nerve
	Finger spreading	Dorsal interossei	Ulnar nerve
T1–T12	Intercostals/respiration	Intercostals	Thoracic and lumbosacral branches
	Trunk muscles	Rectus abdominus and obliques	
L1, 2, 3	Hip flexion	Iliopsoas	Femoral nerve
L2, 3, 4	Knee extension	Quadriceps femoris	Femoral nerve
L4–S2	Foot dorsiflexion	Extensor hallucis and digitorum	Deep peroneal nerve
	Knee flexion	Biceps femoris and hamstrings	Sciatic nerve
L5–S2	Hip extension	Gluteus maximus	Inferior gluteal nerve
L5–S2	Plantar flexion	Gastrocnemius	Tibial nerve

and legs against resistance may be used to evaluate muscle strength. Spontaneous movements should be evaluated in patients who do not follow commands either because of a language deficit or decreased conscious level. Application of painful stimuli may be necessary to elicit sufficient motor responses, such as withdrawal, to determine relative strength of the extremities.

To test the abdominal muscles, ask the patient to flex his or her neck or to sit up from the lying position while the abdominal muscles are palpated. The respiratory musculature is tested by asking the patient to cough, blow out a match, and count while holding his breath.

Contralateral hemiparesis or hemiplegia is characteristic of cerebral hemispheres involvement. Weakness or paralysis associated with peripheral nerve involvement is muscle specific. Spinal cord lesions usually result in bilateral paresis or paralysis below the level of the lesion, and involve not only the muscles of the extremities but also the respiratory and abdominal musculature. Bilateral muscular weakness or paralysis also may be seen in patients with Guillain-Barré syndrome, myasthenia gravis, severe electrolyte disturbances, or systemic toxicity such as botulism.

Muscle Tone

Muscle tone represents the net influence of many complex reflex mechanisms and is reflected by muscle resistance to passive movements. Muscle tone is tested by taking each extremity through a passive range of motion.

Slight resistance is indicative of normal tone. The extremity should move in a smooth, constant, and equal manner throughout the full range.

Decrease or loss of tone (hypotonic or flaccidity) is characterized by limp, flabby muscles and is characteristic of some types of cerebellar dysfunction, the initial period following damage to the cerebral hemispheres or the spinal cord, and peripheral nerve damage.

Increased muscle tone appears as spasticity or rigidity. Spastic muscles have increasing resistance to passive movements and may suddenly give way (clasp-knife phenomenon). Spasticity is indicative of an interruption of the corticospinal (pyramidal) pathways. Interruption of the extrapyramidal system results in muscle rigidity. The muscles may have steadily increasing resistance to passive movement in both flexion and extension (lead-pipe rigidity) as in diffuse brain injury, or may be intermittently and jerkily rigid (cogwheel rigidity) as in Parkinson's.[4]

Posture, whether lying, sitting, or standing, is influenced by muscle strength and maintained by muscle tone. Disturbances of muscle strength and particularly muscle tone result in a wide variety of postural alterations. Some of the most significant postural disturbances occur in patients with altered levels of consciousness.

Coordination

Coordination is primarily under cerebellar control and represents the normal interrelationship between all motor functions of the various muscle groups. Cerebellar testing may be accomplished by asking the patient to perform rapid, rhythmic, alternating movements such as placing the thumb and fingers in apposition, patting his leg as fast as possible with his hand, turning his hand over and back quickly, and tapping the examiner's hand with the ball of his foot. The rapid alternating movements should be smooth, and symmetrical in amplitude and rate. Finger-to-nose and heel-to-knee pointing may be used to demonstrate past-pointing (dysmetria) or intention tremors. The performance on cerebellar testing will be altered by a variety of motor and sensory dysfunctions.

Loss of coordination (ataxia) will be reflected in the patient's ability to speak, swallow, feed, dress, write, maintain trunk balance during sitting and standing, change positions, and walk with a normal gait. Uncoordination may be a result of motor weakness, sensory loss (proprioception and/or vibration), cerebellar and vestibular dysfunction. The specific clinical features of the loss of coordination are directly related to the structural and functional involvement.

Station

Standing, or station, is dependent on motor strength and postural reflexes. The patient should be able to maintain normal equilibrium during standing, with eyes either opened or closed. Ask the patient to stand unsupported with the feet together. Observe his or her ability to maintain an upright position, first with the eyes open and then with them closed. Difficulty standing with the feet together (Romberg's sign) occurs with motor weakness and with proprioceptive, cerebellar, and vestibular dysfunction. In some instances, the patient is able to visually correct and stand erectly, except in the presence of cerebellar dysfunction.[1]

Gait

Gait is the end result of the highly complex mechanisms that achieve motor integration. The ambulatory patient should be observed for a smooth, rhythmic, coordinated gait. He should also be able to walk in a straight line, placing heel to toe (tandem). A wide variety of neurological disorders produce gait abnormalities as well as the total inability to walk, hop in one place, and skip. There are characteristic gait patterns associated with weakness, spasticity, loss of proprioception, and specific cerebellar and basal ganglia diseases.

Involuntary Movements

A comprehensive motor evaluation includes observation of the patient for involuntary muscular movements, which occur in many forms and have a variety of causes.

Tremors are purposeless rhythmic movements of the extremities and/or head. Some of the most common tremors may be described as resting (Parkinsonism), intention (cerebellar), flapping (metabolic encephalopathy), physiologic (stress induced), and senile. *Fasciculations, spasms,* and *tics* are repetitive muscle twitchings that vary slightly in appearance, cause, or site of the pathology. *Clonus* is a repetitive sustained stretch reflex usually seen with the spasticity associated with upper motor neuron lesions.[6] *Seizures* are involuntary motor activities, either generalized or focal, and may be accompanied by loss of awareness for the environment at the time of the seizure and/or muscular contractions of the tonic and/or clonic variety.

SENSORY EXAMINATION

The sensory examination can only be performed satisfactorily with an alert, cooperative, and attentive patient. The reliability also will vary according to the individual patient's intellectual capacity, ability to be objective, and freedom from distractions. Superficial and deep sensation as well as cortical discrimination are included in a comprehensive sensory evaluation. All sensory testing is performed while the patient's eyes are closed.

Superficial Sensations

The superficial sensations include light touch, pain, and temperature. Testing is performed according to the spinal segment dermatomal distribution over the arms, trunk, and legs (See Fig. 1-2). The surface of the skin is stimulated

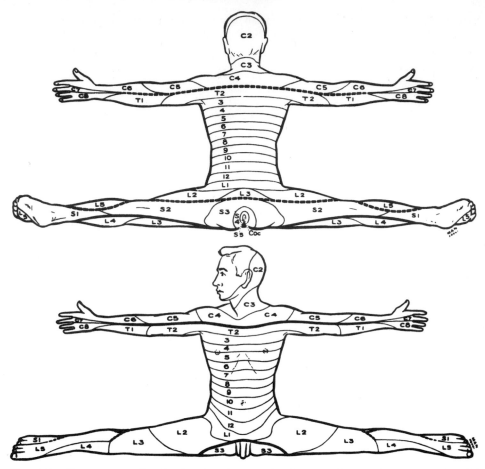

Fig. 1-2. Dermatome distribution for the anterior body surface. (From Haymaker W and Woodhall B: Peripheral Nerve Injuries, 2nd ed., Copyright 1962 by WB Saunders, Philadelphia.)

and the perception of the stimulus is compared in symmetrical areas on each side of the body and between the distal and proximal areas of each extremity. Use a head-to-toe approach and begin in the distal areas of each extremity.

Light touch is tested by using a wisp of cotton, and asking the patient to indicate when he feels the skin is touched. *Pain* is tested by randomly pricking the skin with the blunt and sharp ends of a safety pin. Ask the patient to report whether the sensation is "sharp" or "dull." *Temperature* testing is performed in the same manner using a test tube of ice water and a test tube of hot water. If pain sensation is normal, temperature usually is not tested.[4,6]

Loss of superficial sensation will occur in varying degrees and locations depending on the location of pathology within the central or peripheral nervous systems. Unilateral loss or diminished sensation occurs as a result of peripheral nerve injury or hemisection of the spinal cord. The loss of superficial sensation associated with peripheral nerve injury is ipsilateral, and hemisection of the cord produces contralateral loss.

Deep Sensations

The deeper and more complex sensations include vibration, joint position (proprioception), and deep pressure.

To test *vibratory sense,* a vibrating tuning fork is placed on the bony prominences of the toes, ankles, knees, iliac crest, fingers, wrists, elbows, and spinous processes. The patient should indicate when he feels vibration and when it stops. The examiner stops the tuning fork vibrations at varying time intervals. *Proprioception* is tested by grasping the toes and fingers by the sides of the joints, and moving them up and down. The patient is asked to state which position the toe/finger is pointing when movement is stopped. Stop randomly in both positions and avoid pressure on the upper and lower part of the toe/finger. *Deep pressure/pain* is tested by squeezing the finger joints, the Achilles tendon, the shoulder muscles and/or major extremity muscles.[4,6]

Ipsilateral loss of deep sensation characterizes involvement of the posterior (dorsal) columns of the spinal cord due to trauma, syphillis or peripheral neuropathy.

Cortical Discrimination

Cortical discrimination of sensation represents the ability to interpret superficial and deep sensations at the parietal lobe level. Quality and quantity of sensations are appreciated. Testing is appropriate only in the presence of normal superficial and deep sensory findings. Tests indicative of parietal lobe function include the identification of two-point stimulation, recognition of simultaneous stimulation, number identification, stereognosis, orientation in space, left-right discrimination, and identification of body parts.

Two-point discrimination is tested by using two pins or calipers to stimulate the patient's skin at variable distances. Randomly stimulate using one and two points. Ask the patient to indicate whether he or she feels one or two pin pricks. When the most sensitive areas (e.g., finger tips and lips) are stimulated, the patient will be able to discern two-point stimulation at much closer distances. Simultaneous stimulation is tested by using a pin or a finger to stimulate two corresponding body areas. Alternate between using single and double stimulation. Ask the patient to indicate whether he feels touch on one or both sides of the body. Inability to feel both stimuli is referred to as extinction, or tactile inattention.

Number identification is tested by tracing numbers on the palm of the patient's hands with a sharp pencil. To test *stereognosis* or identification of an object by feeling its shape (without visual clues) place common objects such as a coin, key, and pencil in the patient's hand and request the name or a description of the object.

Orientation in space is tested by asking the patient to indicate with his arm or a stick a vertical, horizontal, and forty-five degree position from the horizontal plane. *Left-right* discrimination is tested by having the patient hold up the left hand and/or identify the left side of a picture of a man. *Identification of body parts* and tactile localization are tested by asking the patient to hold up or point to a specific body part.[4,6]

Loss of cortical discrimination occurs on the contralateral side from the parietal lobe lesion. A thalamic lesion produces loss of all contralateral bodily sensations plus the presence of severe spontaneous pain on the same side as the deficits.

REFLEXES

Reflexes are involuntary motor responses to sensory stimuli. Interruption of the impulse transmission along the reflex arc will result in loss of the appropriate motor response. Reflexes are under the influence of brainstem, cerebral, and cerebellar structures, which either facilitate or inhibit the motor response. Motor responses may be either absent (areflexic), diminished, normal, or exaggerated. Pathologic reflexes occur with cortical damage and when reflex centers are separated from their upper motor neuron connections.[7]

There are three major types of reflexes: superficial (skin and mucous membrane), deep tendon (stretch), and pathologic (abnormal). Examples of superficial reflexes involving the mucous membranes include the gag and corneal reflexes, which are evaluated during the cranial nerve examination.

Superficial Reflexes

Major superficial skin reflexes include the abdominal, the cremasteric, the plantar, and the anal reflexes. The *abdominal reflexes* are tested by stimulating each quadrant of the abdomen with a moderately sharp object above and below the umbilicus while the patient is lying down. Normally the muscles contract when stimulated and the umbilicus moves toward the stimulated side. Inability of the patient to relax or obesity will make the reflex difficult to elicit. Absence of the reflex is indicative of an upper motor neuron lesion at or above the level of T8–12 segments. The *cremasteric reflex* is tested by stroking the inner surface of the thigh to produce elevation of the testicle on the same side. Loss of the reflex is indicative of an upper motor neuron lesion at or above the L1–2 segments.

The *plantar reflex* is tested by stroking the lateral aspect of the sole of the foot with a blunt object, e.g., a key. As the key is moved along the sole toward the little toe and around to the big toe, the toes normally flex. Extension of

Table 1-2.

Reflex	Spinal Segment	Normal Response
Biceps	C5–6	Elbow flexion
Triceps	C6–8	Elbow extension
Wrist (brachioradialis)	C6–8	Wrist extension
Knee (patellar)	L2–4	Knee extension
Ankle (Achilles)	S1–2	Foot extension

the big toe with flaring of the small toes (Babinski sign) is indicative of upper motor neuron lesions. The *anal reflex* is tested by stroking the skin around the anus and perineum with a pin, or placing a gloved finger in the rectum. Either method normally produces contraction of the anal sphincter. Loss of this reflex occurs with damage at or above the S3–5 spinal cord segment level.[3,6]

Deep Tendon Reflexes

The deep tendon or stretch reflexes are elicited by briskly tapping the point of muscle insertion with a reflex hammer and observing the resultant muscle contraction. The patient needs to be relaxed to permit the appropriate response. Symmetrically diminished or absent reflexes may be due to poor relaxation. The patient may be asked to isometrically contract other muscles, e.g., clench teeth, lock fingers together and pull one hand against the other. This technique is called reinforcement and should facilitate reflex response. The most common deep tendon reflexes tested are biceps, triceps, brachioradialis, quadriceps, and Achilles tendon. Table 1-2 identifies the spinal cord segment involved and the normal response.

Deep tendon reflexes will be lost or diminished in the presence of primary reflex pathway pathology. Hyperactive reflexes are characteristic of upper motor neuron lesions.

Pathologic Reflexes

Pathologic reflexes characteristic of cortical damage include the glabella, snout, sucking, chewing, and grasp. Many are primitive reflexes that are normal in the infant. Persistance or reappearance of these reflexes in the older child or adult indicates loss of frontal lobe inhibitory functions.

The *glabella* is elicited by tapping the forehead between the eyebrows with a finger. Persistent, spasmodic closure of the eyelids in indicative of frontal lobe dysfunction. The *snout reflex* is an excessive grimace of the face in response to tapping the nose. This is characteristic of bilateral corticopontine lesions. Stroking the lips with a finger or with a tongue blade will elicit pouting and *sucking* movements in the presence of frontal lobe lesions. Reflex chewing movements on a tongue depressor is called the *chewing reflex*. The jaw may be clamped so tightly that the tongue blade may be difficult to remove. Reflex chewing is characteristic of bilateral frontal pathology. Stroking the palm of the patient's hand may elicit a firm grip on the examiner's hand. This is called the *grasp reflex*. It may be very difficult for the examiner to remove his or her hand from a firm grasp reflex.[3]

ASSESSMENT OF PATIENTS WITH ALTERED STATES OF CONSCIOUSNESS

Acute alteration of consciousness may occur as a consequence of structural damage to the cerebral hemispheres and/or brainstem reticular formation, or diffuse metabolic encephalopathy. The structural damage may be ischemic, hemorrhagic, or compressive in origin. The site of structural damage may be supratentorial, infratentorial, or diffuse. The common causes of metabolic cerebral dysfunction include hypoxia, ischemia, hypoglycemia, water/sodium imbalance, acid/base imbalance, liver or kidney disease, sepsis, and exogenous poisons (e.g., sedatives, alcohol, and psychotropic drugs).[8]

Consciousness reflects the functional integrity of the brain as a whole. Although conscious level is a very sensitive index of brain dysfunction, other physiologic variables provide the information required to identify the extent, location, and nature of intracranial pathology, and to determine whether the patient is improving or deteriorating. Therefore, the key parameters in the assessment of neurologic status include conscious level, pupillary activity, ocular movements, respiratory pattern, and blood pressure/pulse rate.[8] The frequency of the neurologic assessment will depend on the acuity of the patient's condition, and the rapidity with which changes are occurring or may be expected.

Conscious Level

Consciousness is awareness of the self and the environment. An individual's state of consciousness is reflected by his or her ability to be aroused, to perceive environmental stimuli, and to respond appropriately on a cognitive and motor level. The stimulus may be internally or externally generated. The responses may be altered by focal sensory and/or motor deficits.

Arousability depends on the integrity of the reticular activating system (RAS), a network of nuclei that form a central core in the brainstem and extend to the thalamic nuclei within the cerebral hemispheres. Cognitive ability depends on the integrity of the cerebral cortex. The complex feedback mechanisms between the RAS and the cerebral cortex permit reciprocal stimulation and modulation of conscious behavior.[8]

Coma is the total absence of awareness of self and environment, even in the presence of external stimulation. There are various degrees of altered states between consciousness and coma. The levels will be dependent on the distribution and extent of the pathological processes.

An objective assessment of conscious level consists of systematically determining the type and degree of external stimuli required to produce a patient response. The stimulus may be verbal, tactile, and/or noxious. The responses must be evaluated in terms of the appropriateness to the situation. When applying stimuli, it is important to arouse the patient maximally before evaluating the quality of the responses. Conscious level is best reflected by eye opening, verbalizations, and arm movements. Each type of response may be initiated voluntarily by the patient or may be reflex in nature.

Responses in the category of *eye opening* include spontaneous response, to speech, to pain, and no response. Spontaneous eye opening may occur as the nurse approaches the bedside. Calling the patient by name, requesting that he open his eyes, or applying a painful stimulus may elicit opening of one or both eyes. It is important to differentiate between eye opening as a response to sound or to a specific command. Spontaneous blinking or a response to sound suggests that the pontine reticular formation is intact. There may be total absence of eye opening regardless of the type of stimulation. The absence of bilateral eye opening is usually indicative of severe depression of the RAS. Consideration must be given to the fact that oculomotor paralysis or eye trauma may prevent appropriate eye opening even in response to pain.

Acute alterations of consciousness have associated tonic eyelid closure. The eyelids close gradually after being opened and released. Significant resistance to eye opening or rapid closure may occur in the presence of both structural and metabolic dysfunction. The eyes may remain open without spontaneous blinking and open gradually after manual closure when there is severe brainstem involvement; this should not be confused with spontaneous eye opening.

Responses in the category of *verbalization* include oriented, confused conversation, inappropriate words, incomprehensible sounds, and no responses. An oriented patient is one who gives accurate information as to the year and month, who he is, where he is, where he lives, and other personal data. A patient who has confused conversation is able to produce language, but unable to give all the correct answers to questions of orientation. Memory for recent and past events, as well as immediate recall, may be impaired and therefore influence the patient's orientation. Inappropriate words may represent dysphasia or the words obtained by physical stimulation rather than verbal stimulation. In this situation, there is no sustained conversation and the words are disorganized or inappropriate. They may take the form of swearing. Incomprehensible sounds consist of moans, groans, and indistinct mumblings. The lowest level of response may be an absence of sound even to painful stimulation; however, this will also occur when there is an endotracheal tube or a tracheostomy in place.

Cortical dysfunction is characterized by confusion and language disturbances, particularly with involvement of the left hemisphere. Corticobulbar dysfunction will interfere with the ability to produce sounds. RAS depression interferes with the ability to appreciate sensory input and therefore make appropriate verbal responses.

Responses in the category of *best motor responses* (in the upper extremities) include obeys commands, localizes pain, withdrawal from pain, flexion to pain, extension to pain, and no response to pain. The patient is expected to perform specific tasks upon verbal or written command or gestures as an indication of motor responsiveness. These commands may include "stick out your tongue," "raise your arms," "hold up two fingers," and "squeeze and release my fingers." If there is no response to commands, painful stimuli should be applied and the specific responses evaluated. Pinch the external ear, the trapezius muscle, or the back of the neck to apply painful stimuli. Do not pinch the skin as it may result in undue trauma and bruising. If the patient localizes pain, he will reach purposefully in an attempt to locate the painful stimulus and remove it. If there is no localized response, apply pressure to the fingernail bed to elicit withdrawal by a normal flexing of the arm.[9] Loss of arousability and depressed consciousness will decrease the effectiveness of motor responses to command and to pain; however, appropriate avoidance responses will remain as long as the RAS and the cortical connections are intact. It is imperative not to confuse focal paralysis or a language barrier with a depressed conscious level.

Abnormal motor responses include flexor and extensor posturing, and flaccidity. Flexor and extensor posturing may occur as an inappropriate response to pain or may appear spontaneously as a result of internally generated stimuli, e.g., pain or distended bladder. Flexor posturing (decorticate rigidity) consists of flexion and adduction of the arm, wrist, and fingers. Extensor posture (decerebrate rigidity) consists of arm extension, adduction, and internal rotation. The fully developed flexor and extensor postures include leg extension, internal rotation, and plantar flexion. Flexor and extensor responses correlate with functional and structural impairment of cortical and subcortical regions of the brain and with the severity of the impairment. There is a loss of cortical inhibitory influence over deep hemispheric and upper brainstem motor tracts when flexor and extensor posturing occurs. Flexor responses reflect less extensive hemispheric involvement without brainstem disruption and a less severe prognosis. Extensor posture is frequently associated with bilateral hemispheric structural damage (diencephalon) or severe metabolic disorders. Clinically, there may be alternation between flexor and extensor posturing or a combination of both, depending on the effect of pressure and blood flow to the upper brainstem. The absence of detectable movement or changes in muscle tone (flaccidity) due to intracranial pathology is characteristic of significant depression of the central motor mechanisms in the brainstem.[8]

Pupillary Activity

Pupil size and reactivity have localizing value and provide clues to the cause of altered states of consciousness. The parasympathetic pathways, which control pupil constriction, follow the course of the oculomotor nerve as it passes over the medial edge of the tentorium in the midbrain. The sympathetic pupil innervators, which produce pupil dilatation, originate in the hypothalamus and descend within the brainstem. Pupil dilatation is also under the influence of the frontal and occipital lobes. The pupil size represents a balance between the two types of innervation. Unopposed innervation results in a predominance of either pupil constriction or dilatation, as seen in destructive lesions. Irritative lesions result in an excessive response from overstimulation. The pupillary pathways are relatively resistant to metabolic influence. Therefore pupil equality and the light reflexes are significant in the determination of structurally versus metabolically induced depression of conscious level.

Posterior and ventrolateral hypothalamic damage is characterized by ipsilateral pupil constriction and is usually associated with ptosis and anhidrosis involving the ipsilateral half of the body (Horner's syndrome). Downward hypothalamic displacement results in a unilateral Horner's syndrome, which may precede transtentorial herniation.[8] Herniation of the uncus of the temporal lobe over the edge of the tentorium results in an ipsilateral nonreactive pupil and dilated pupil due to pressure on the parasympathetic fibers of the oculomotor nerve. Symmetrically small pupils are associated with central supratentorial mass lesions and metabolic encephalopathies. Bilateral pinpoint pupils are consistent with pontine lesions and the use of opiates.

Midbrain damage results in loss of the pupil light reflex but the response to accommodation may be preserved. The pupils are midposition, light fixed, show hippus (alternate constriction and dilatation) and an intact ciliospinal reflex. The light reflex remains intact with metabolic encephalopathies.

Involvement of the oculomotor nuclei is characterized by bilaterally dilated, nonreactive pupils. Involvement of the peripheral portion of the oculomotor nerve results in ipsilateral pupil dilatation and loss of the light reflex, as is seen in tentorial herniation. Dilated pupils may be a temporary consequence of major motor seizure activity. Bilaterally dilated pupils are characteristic of the intake of large quantities of atropine, scopolamine, barbiturate intoxication, severe hypoxia or ischemia, circulatory arrest, and brain death.[8]

Ocular Movements

Ocular movements are controlled by the third, fourth, and sixth cranial nerves as well as by brainstem pathways, which are adjacent to the RAS and under the influence of the cerebral hemispheres. The movements may be spontaneous and reflexive in nature. The eye movements and the presence or absence of the oculocephalic (dolls eye) and oculovestibular (caloric) reflexes provide information regarding the integrity of the brainstem, the location of the pathology, and the potential for altered respiratory function, particularly in the patient with an altered state of consciousness.

Patients with depressed levels of consciousness frequently demonstrate spontaneous, roving, random eye movements which may be conjugate or dysconjugate. The eye movement may be repetitive and rhythmic. The roving movements tend to disappear with significant depression of brainstem activity, regardless of the cause. Dysconjugate eye movement is very characteristic of structural damage to the brainstem whereas hemispheric damage usually results in conjugate deviation. Destructive lesions of a hemisphere are characterized by lateral deviation of the eyes to the same side as the cerebral lesion. Lateral deviation to the opposite side is consistent with an irritative cerebral lesion. Eye deviation toward the paralyzed side suggests a pontine brainstem lesion. The localizing value of eye movements in patients with altered states of consciousness is complimented by the ocular reflex testing.[5,8]

The oculocephalic (doll's eye) reflex is elicited by holding the eyelids of an unresponsive patient open and briskly rotating the head from one side to the other, pausing briefly on each side. The normal response is conjugate deviation to the opposite side. Brisk flexion and extension of the neck results in deviation of the eyes up or down, respectively. As the neck is flexed, the eyelids may open reflexively. The eyes should return to resting position a few seconds after each maneuver, regardless of the position of the head. The oculovestibular (caloric) reflex is elicited by slowly irrigating the external auditory canal with approximately 100 cc of ice water. When consciousness is depressed, the normal response is conjugate eye deviation toward the irrigated ear.

The responses to stimulation by passive head turning and ice water are related to each other, differing only in degree. Generally, oculovestibular stimulation is stronger than oculocephalic stimulation. In the presence of cortical depression and an intact brainstem, both reflexes will be brisk and appropriate. Massive hemispheric damage may interfere with the ability to produce normal ocular responses even though the brainstem is intact due to the strong eye deviation toward the damaged hemisphere. Brainstem destruction or compression produces abnormal responses to both types of stimulation. Midbrain compression results in loss of reflex upward gaze. Unilateral involvement of the oculomotor or abducens nuclei or nerves results in loss of the responses to the ipsilateral side. Bilateral brainstem lesions result in the inability to deviate the eyes across the midline in either direction. Lower brainstem lesions interfere with the normal responses in both the lateral and vertical plane.[5,8]

Reflex eye movements will remain intact with metabolically induced cerebral depression; however, the movements will become sluggish and finally disappear with severe brainstem depression from a sedative overdose. The oculocephalic reflex is particularly sensitive to depressant drugs and therefore will disappear before the oculovestibular reflex. Although intact ocular reflexes imply structural integrity of the brainstem, the absence of these reflexes does not confirm loss of brainstem function nor does it identify the cause of the loss of consciousness.[8]

Respiratory Pattern

Respirations represent a highly integrated activity that is influenced by a variety of cerebral, brainstem, upper cervical cord, and metabolic control mechanisms. The principal site of integration occurs in the lower brainstem. Patients with a depressed conscious level frequently have concomitant alterations in respiratory function. The breathing pattern represents the most significant respiratory parameter that changes in the presence of neurological deterioration. There is a close correlation between the characteristics of the respiratory pattern and the level of involvement of the brain and brainstem.[8] There are both therapeutic and prognostic implications associated with the various abnormal patterns.

The variety of abnormal respiratory patterns represents dysfunction of the pontine centers which facilitate hyperventilation; dysfunction of the cerebral centers which exert inhibitory control over the pontine centers; and the metabolic influence of the chemoreceptors in the carotid body, aortic wall, and lower brainstem which respond to CO_2 tension and pH changes. The most common respiratory patterns that occur in patients with alteration of conscious level from structurally or metabolically induced depression include Cheyne-

Stokes respirations, central neurogenic hyperventilation, apneustic breathing, cluster breathing, and ataxic breathing. For more information regarding these respiratory patterns and the associated intracranial pathology see the chapter on "Respiratory Complications of Intracranial Disorders."

Patients with altered states of consciousness from neurological involvement are highly susceptible to further damage and deterioration in the presence of inadequate pulmonary function and oxygenation. In addition to the recognition of the characteristic respiratory patterns and the implications of each, a variety of other respiratory parameters are essential to overall patient management. In addition to assessment of respiratory patterns, a comprehensive evaluation of respiratory function must include rate, arterial oxygen and carbon dioxide tensions, breath sounds, the ability of the patient to breath spontaneously, maintain a patent airway, cough, and handle oral secretions. Dysfunction in one or a combination of these respiratory activities may be a direct result of structural brain damage or metabolic encephalopathy.

Blood Pressure/Pulse Rate

The alterations in blood pressure, heart rate, and rhythm, which occur in patients with intracranial pathology, are usually associated with increased intracranial pressure or a secondary cardiovascular instability. The classic cardiovascular response (Cushing's reflex) to sustained increases in intracranial pressure include an increase in systolic blood pressure, a widening pulse pressure, and bradycardia. The blood pressure is controlled by nuclei in the medulla. As the medulla becomes compressed and ischemic from the increase in intracranial pressure, there is a concomitant increase in cardiac output which is reflected as an increase in systolic pressure. The increase in cardiac output is the result of an increase in heart rate. As the pulse pressure widens, the baroreceptors are stimulated, producing a vagal response (bradycardia). The Cushing's reflex occurs late in the herniation process and usually implies significant brainstem compromise. However, it is an unreliable sign because it only occurs in a small percentage of patients.

The cardiac rate, rhythm, and systemic blood pressure are under the influence of a variety of hemispheric, hypothalamic, and brainstem structures along with their descending pathways. The specific cardiovascular abnormality depends on the location of the damage. Hypertension, hypotension, and disturbances of cardiac rate, rhythm, and electrical activity may be neurogenic in origin. Monitoring of blood pressure is not utilized as a diagnostic tool, but gains significance in the management of patients with altered states of consciousness. The ECG abnormalities or dysrhythmias correlate with cerebrovascular disorders, e.g., subarachnoid hemorrhage and acute stroke. Acute intracranial bleeding may precipitate massive, brief autonomic discharges from the sudden increase in the intracranial pressure. The abnormal ECG findings may include conduction defects, PVCs, tachycardia, bradycardia, and arrest[8] (see chapter on "Cardiovascular Complications of Intracranial Disorders").

Motor Function

The neurological evaluation of patients with altered states of consciousness will vary considerably from the evaluation of alert patients. The motor and reflex evaluation of patients with depression of conscious level will assist in defining structural versus metabolic problems, identification of neurological deterioration, and provide direction for the appropriate patient management. However, depression of the conscious level requires modification of the techniques used to determine the functional deficits.

Determination of the presence or absence of symmetrical muscle strength, tone, and reflex activity are important to compliment the motor findings, which are used as an index of conscious level. The deficits may be bilateral in the presence of diffuse nervous system involvement or unilateral as a result of focal damage or irritation. Loss of muscle strength and/or tone are reflected by facial asymmetry, inability to grimace in response to pain, the resting position of the head and extremities, and lack of spontaneous movement. An extremity that has lost strength and tone will drop limply when picked up and released. Muscle tone will slow the fall and promote anatomical alignment. Types of increased tone such as paratonia, gegenhalten, or resistance to passive movements of the head, trunk, and extremities disappear as the body part is moved slowly, and becomes exaggerated as the part is moved rapidly.

Patients with altered states of consciousness should be evaluated for the absence of the protective reflexes and the reappearance of primitive or infantile reflex activities. The presence of spontaneous blinking and swallowing should be noted. Absence of blinking to a threat (menace reflex) suggests visual impairment, particularly when there is spontaneous eye closure. Decreased spontaneous swallowing and an inability to handle oral secretions suggests an impaired gag reflex or a very depressed level of consciousness. Grasp, sucking, and snout reflex responses frequently accompany altered states of consciousness when the frontal lobes are damaged.

CONCLUSION

The nurse has a primary responsibility for the accurate, knowledgeable assessment of all parameters that are significant in determining changes in the patient's clinical status. There must be anticipation, prevention, recognition, reporting, and recording of all deviations in function. Different disease processes involving the nervous system may produce an identical clinical picture. Conversely, a specific disease may produce a wide variation in the clinical presentation. Nervous system dysfunction is usually a very dynamic process. The quality of patient care and the type of management will be greatly influenced by the skill of the nursing personnel evaluating subtle changes in the patients clinical status.

REFERENCES

1. Alpers B and Mancell E: Essentials of the Neurological Examination. 2nd ed. FA Davis, Philadelphia, 1981.
2. Wallhagen MI: The split brain: Implications for care and rehabilitation, American Journal of Nursing 79:2118, 1979.
3. Chusid Joseph G: Correlative Neuroanatomy and Functional Neurology. 17th Ed. Lange Medical Publications, Los Altos, California, 1979.
4. Gilroy J and Meyer JS: Medical Neurology. 3rd Ed. Macmillan, New York, 1979.
5. Wolf J: Practical Clinical Neurology. Medical Examination Publishing Company, New York, 1980.
6. Bates Barbara: A Guide to Physical Examination. 2nd Ed. JB Lippincott, Philadelphia, 1979.
7. DeMyer W: Technique of the Neurological Examination. McGraw-Hill, New York, 1980.
8. Plum F and Posner J: The Diagnosis of Stupor and Coma. 3rd Ed. FA Davis, Philadelphia, 1980.
9. Teasdale G: Acute impairment of brain function: Assessing conscious level. Nursing Times 71:914, 1975.

2 | Intracranial Pressure: Dynamics, Assessment, and Control

Pamela H. Mitchell

Intracranial hypertension—increased intracranial pressure (ICP)—is a serious and potentially fatal complication of a variety of neurologic conditions affecting the critically ill patient. The advent of continuous monitoring of ICP has led to an exponential increase in knowledge of the physiology of the condition and of methods to control or reduce intracranial hypertension.

Important nursing and medical goals in the patient at risk for intracranial hypertension are 1) early detection of intracranial hypertension; 2) reduction of ICP to levels that permit adequate brain perfusion; and 3) prevention of transient and sustained increases of ICP in patients with existing intracranial hypertension.

The purpose of this chapter is to describe the processes that undergird the achievement of those goals. The concepts and processes include determinants of normal intracranial pressure, the pathophysiology of intracranial hypertension, and methods to detect and control intracranial hypertension in the critically ill patient.

Elevated intracranial pressure is not dangerous in itself. All of us experience transient increase in ICP when we cough, sneeze, or when we strain while eliminating stool. Compensatory measures quickly reduce ICP before blood flow to neurons is compromised. The critically ill patient with a neurologic disorder who experiences increased ICP is at serious risk of compromised cerebral function for several reasons: brain cells are already damaged or ischemic from the primary injury, compensatory mechanisms may be impaired by the primary disease process, and cerebral blood flow may be altered. Consequently, changes in ICP that may be of no consequence in the healthy brain may impose further damage on an already impaired brain.

THE DYNAMICS OF MAINTAINING INTRACRANIAL PRESSURE

Intracranial pressure normally varies between 0 and 10 torr.* Oscillations in pressure occur with respiratory cycles, and more rapid oscillations occur with each cardiac cycle. The shape of the intracranial pulse wave, measured in the ventricular fluid, is the same as that of the blood pressure waveform.

Intracranial pressure is most accurately measured from the cerebral ventricles, as ventricular fluid pressure (VFP). Lumbar cerebrospinal fluid (CSF) pressure is equal to VFP in the recumbent position, provided that there is free communication of CSF from brain to spinal dural sac.[1] In patients with neural trauma or disease, it is likely that such free communication is not present and that lumbar measurements will not reflect those of the cranial cavity. Furthermore, if pressure in the cranial cavity is higher than in the spinal cavity, and if CSF is subsequently withdrawn from the lumbar space, the pressure differential can cause herniation of the brain into the foramen magnum, and death.[2]

Factors Maintaining Normal ICP

For well over a hundred years it has been known that the intracranial pressure is dependent upon the relationships among the three components of the cranial cavity: the brain, the blood, and the cerebrospinal fluid. The cranial cavity may be considered as an almost closed box, slightly vented via the venous system. As a nearly closed box, the volume within must remain essentially constant or pressure will rise. It follows then that if the volume of any one of the three components increases, the volume of the other two must be displaced or ICP will rise.

As shown in Fig. 2-1, when additional volume is added to the intracranial cavity, pressure does not rise initially. At a given point, however (Fig. 2-1, arrow), pressure begins to rise exponentially with the addition of the same volume that previously produced no change. The flat portion of the curve may then be considered a stage in which the intracranial volumes are adjusting to maintain equilibrium in intracranial pressure. The steep portion of the curve represents a state of decompensation in which very small changes in intracranial volume will produce large changes in pressure.[1,3] Theoretically, any of three volumes could be altered to accommodate change in intracranial volume. In fact, the CSF provides the major buffer to change in intracranial volume.[1,4,5]

---

* Torr is a unit of pressure equivalent to millimeters of Hg. 1 torr = 1 mm Hg.

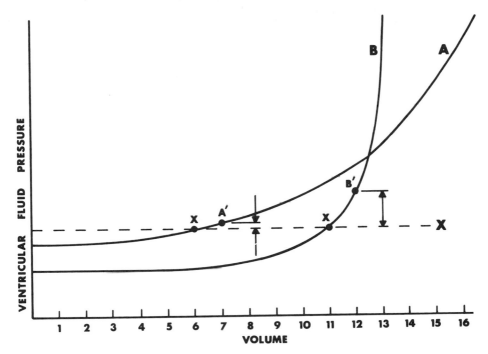

Fig. 2-1. Two theoretical volume–pressure curves in different patients. At the same resting pressure (X), addition of 1 unit of volume produces a greater pressure increase on the B curve than the A curve (B′ > A′). From: N. Mauss and P. Mitchell: Increased intracranial pressure: an update, Heart and Lung 5:920, 1976. Used by permission of the authors and publisher.

Displacement of CSF. Cerebrospinal fluid is produced in the choroid plexus of the cerebral ventricles, passes from the lateral ventricles downward to the third and fourth ventricles, and then out through the foramen of Magendie and Luschka (the basal cisterns). CSF then passes both upward (to be absorbed over the convexities of the brain) and downward into the spinal dural sac. The spinal sac acts as a capacitance vessel, holding approximately 140 ml compared to the 20–30 ml found in the ventricles.[6] When intracranial volume increases, more CSF is expressed into the spinal sac, which can expand considerably.[7] In addition, a small increase in absorption of CSF in both brain and spinal cord is seen with increased ICP.[1]

Reduction in Cerebral Blood Volume. A second compensatory response to an increase in intracranial volume is the displacement of some blood into the venous sinuses.[1,4] This mechanism cannot displace so large a volume as the CSF buffering system, and is best visualized as the sloping portion of the volume-pressure curve (Fig. 2-1).

Displacement of Brain Tissue. Expansion of brain volume, with a tumor, hemorrhage, or edema, for example, is the most common cause of expanding intracranial volume. The brain is often considered relatively noncompressible. However, with slowly growing intracranial volumes, the brain does exhibit some ability to be compressed. The steep portion of each curve in Fig. 2-1 represents the elasticity or ability to resist compression of the brain. With rapidly expanding intracranial volume, as shown in curve B in Fig. 2-1, there is an almost linear relationship between addition of volume and elasticity of the brain. In other words, the brain does not compress to compensate for the added volume. If the brain herniates through the tentorium or foramen magnum, a new equilibrium is reached and the curve will flatten once again. Such a compensatory mechanism is obviously fatal to the patient.

The volume-pressure curve for a more slowly growing lesion, for example, a brain tumor, would resemble curve A in Fig. 2-1. In such a curve, the slope is not so steep and suggests that the brain is more elastic, and that compression of tissue may have occurred.[8] This deformation and compression of brain tissue is seen with such disorders as chronic subdural hematoma and encapsulated tumors.

Volume-Pressure Relationships

The relationships between volume and pressure in the craniospinal cavities can be quantified and used clinically to estimate the status on the curve of any given patient. The relationship of a change in volume to a change in pressure (dV/dP) is called compliance and is most appropriately applied to the flat portion of the curve in which changes in CSF volume are occurring in response to change in pressure. Change in pressure related to change in volume (dP/dV) is called elastance and is exemplified by the steep portion of the curve in which small changes in volume (usually cerebral blood volume or trapped CSF) produce large changes in pressure.[9] These relationships may be quantified by the volume-pressure response (VPR) of Miller[10] or the pressure-volume index (PVI) of Marmarou.[11] Methods of calculating these indices are discussed later.

The clinical importance of understanding volume-pressure relationships is twofold. First, if one understands the concept of compliance/elastance it is possible to explain why the same care activity, for example, suctioning, may produce a large change in ICP in one patient and not in another, even though both have the same resting ICP. The patient who shows a large change can be presumed to have exhausted compensatory volume displacement mechanisms, and has a volume-pressure relationship on the steep part of the curve. In contrast, the patient who shows little or no change may still be able to displace CSF into the spinal cavity, or blood into the venous system. Thus, one cannot predict the response of any given patient to any activity that results in adding volume to the cranial cavity by knowing only the resting ICP level.

Secondly, once compensatory measures have been exhausted, any further changes in intracranial volume result in very large changes in ICP. Thus, patients with high elastance (volume-pressure relationship on the steep portion of the curve) may experience large and potentially dangerous increases in ICP with ordinary activities of daily living, or nursing care maneuvers that were previously of little consequence.

INTRACRANIAL HYPERTENSION

When the ability of the cranial-spinal cavity to displace volume has reached capacity, ICP begins to rise, and will rise sharply with further additions to intracranial volume. When mean ICP is elevated to 15 torr and beyond, intracranial hypertension exists.* Miller and colleagues recommend considering mean ICP that is greater than 10 torr to be elevated.[12] This recommendation is based on the observation that the range of ICP between 10 and 15 torr contains those persons who have "normal" resting pressures but high elastance (large change in pressure with small change in volume).

As stated earlier, intracranial hypertension *in itself* is not harmful. However, it becomes dangerous in the injured brain when it is sufficiently high to reduce cerebral perfusion pressure (CPP) to critical levels.

The CPP necessary to maintain brain function varies with the state of metabolism of the brain. In normal brains, CPP may fall as low as 20–30 torr without evidence of neurophysiological dysfunction, although blood flow falls to about 50 percent of normal.[13] Patients with benign intracranial hypertension (pseudotumor cerebri) may tolerate very low CPP without apparent harm.[14] However, patients with injured brains may have areas of very high metabolism, as well as disordered mechanisms regulating blood flow. In such persons, EEG and other functional changes are seen with CPP less than 40–50 torr.[15,16] Therefore, most authorities recommend maintaining CPP of at least 50 torr in such critically ill patients.

Factors Affecting Intracranial Volume in the Patient with Intracranial Hypertension

In states of disease and trauma, brain volume will increase through such events as tumor growth, cerebral edema or intracranial hemorrhage (extradural, subdural, or intracerebral). Cerebral blood volume may change with increases in cerebral blood flow, vasodilatation, or obstruction of venous outflow.

The volume of cerebrospinal fluid can increase through increased production, decreased reabsorption, or obstruction of outflow to the basal cisterns or to the spinal cavity.

Brain Volume. Pathologic states that act to increase brain mass are common causes of intracranial hypertension in the critically ill person. These include rapidly growing tumors; epidural, subdural, and intracerebral hematomas following trauma; hypertensive intracerebral bleeding; abscesses that act as masses; and focal or general cerebral edema.

Cerebral edema is best defined as any increase in the water content of the

---

* Mean ICP is estimated in the same manner as mean arterial blood pressure

$$\bar{X}ICP = \frac{systolic\ ICP - diastolic\ ICP}{3} + diastolic\ ICP$$

brain.[17-19] Vascular engorgement, without an increase in brain water, is considered later, under "Blood Volume." Either focal or general cerebral edema can lead to increased ICP if the water content of the brain expands sufficiently to overcome compensatory changes in the volume of CSF or blood in the cranium.

Vasogenic, cytotoxic, hydrostatic, and osmotic forces can act to produce cerebral edema. In contrast to peripheral edema, brain edema can be either extracellular or intracellular, or combinations of both. Brain capillaries are surrounded by epithelial basement membrane and by the foot processes of astrocytes. These membrane and astrocytic processes form what are known as "tight junctions." The relative impermeability of these junctions to the passage of large molecules is thought to be the basis of the blood-brain barrier. Vascular damage disrupts these junctions and allows large molecules, e.g., proteins, to slip from the capillary into the interstitial spaces of the brain. In addition, such damage may allow the movement of ions and molecules by pinocytosis, a process not seen in the normal brain.[18] Water follows these molecules to maintain osmotic equilibrium and protein-rich edema fluid collects in the interstitial space. This *vasogenic* edema is found clinically surrounding tumors, abscesses, and contusions.

Water will collect interstitially in *hydrostatic* edema, but the fluid is not protein-rich. Such edema occurs when high intravascular pressures are not balanced by an increase in cerebrovascular resistance. Water extravasates into the extracellular spaces by hydrostatic force alone. Profound hypertension, trauma, hypercapnia, and profound hypoxia can lead to these sudden shifts in Starling forces.* In addition, the sudden brain swelling sometimes seen with surgical decompression may represent hydrostatic edema.[18]

A final source of extracellular edema is the accumulation of CSF around the ventricles as seen in chronic hydrocephalus. This has been termed *interstitial* edema.[17]

Intracellular accumulations of fluid occur in *cytotoxic* and *hypoosmotic* edema.[18] Some authorities classify all clinical edema caused by hypoxia, cell poisoning, and hypoosmolarity as of the cytotoxic type.[17,19] In edema of this type, the tight junctions around the capillaries remain intact, but the metabolic machinery of the glial cells breaks down. Sodium accumulates within the cell and water enters to maintain osmotic equilibrium. Astrocytes in particular are subject to this intracellular swelling. Clinically such edema is seen in Reye's syndrome, cerebral hypoxia, and hypoosmolar syndromes (acute water intoxication, inappropriate ADH secretion).

While cytotoxic-type edemas may be seen clinically in relatively pure form, the extracellular edemas often produce cellular hypoxia-ischemia and thus have concomitant cytotoxic components.

---

* Starling forces are those governing passage of water across capillary membranes: capillary hydrostatic pressure + tissue colloid osmotic pressure = tissue hydrostatic pressure + plasma colloid osmotic pressure.

Blood Volume.   Marked increase in cerebral blood flow and volume through loss of autoregulation can be a major factor inducing intracranial hypertension in injured brains. Furthermore, when intracranial hypertension already exists, and when elastance is high, even small increases in cerebral blood volume can produce large increases in ICP. Such increases in blood volume can occur through increases in systemic blood pressure, vasodilatation of cerebral vessels, and obstruction of venous outflow.

Fluctuations in Blood Pressure.   Normally, cerebral vessels dilate and constrict as necessary to maintain a constant cerebral blood flow, regardless of fluctuations in systemic blood pressure. This phenomenon is known as autoregulation. Thus, in the normal person, fluctuations in mean arterial blood pressure between about 50 and 150 torr do not alter cerebral blood flow.[20] Mean arterial blood pressures at either extreme of the range "break through" autoregulation and may decrease or increase CBF, respectively. In the injured brain, however, autoregulation may not be intact due to metabolic changes, or may function within a much narrower range. In such situations, normal fluctuations in systemic blood pressure may be directly reflected in increased or decreased cerebral blood flow. Large changes in blood pressure can occur with many activities such as straining during elimination, pushing oneself up or down in bed, decerebrate and decorticate posturing, and during coughing or suctioning.

Vasodilatation.   Hypercarbia, profound hypoxia, and certain volatile anesthetics can produce vasodilatation in the critically ill person. Hypercarbia produces the most dramatic changes in cerebral vessel size, almost on a mm for mm basis.[21] Any situation that results in retention of secretions or impairment of respiratory drive can create hypercarbia in the critically ill patient.

Cerebral blood vessels do not respond by vasodilatation to changes in arterial oxygen until PaO_2 is about 50 torr and lower.[22,23] PaO_2 can easily drop to these levels during suctioning.[24,25]

The anesthetic agents most often implicated in increasing cerebral blood volume through vasodilatation are halothane, nitrous oxide, and ketamine.[26] For this reason, these drugs are rarely used in neuroanesthesia.

Obstruction of Venous Outflow.   The final mechanism altering cerebral blood volume is obstruction to venous outflow. One of the compensatory mechanisms during increasing cerebral volume is a shift of blood to the cerebral venous system. Once this system has reached capacity, any small decrease in outflow, through obstruction of major or collateral venous channels, will "trap" blood in the cranial cavity and increase cerebral blood volume.

Arterial blood in the brain passes via the capillaries to the venous system, collects in the superior sagittal sinus, and drains primarily through the internal jugular vein. Secondary outflow channels include the vertebral veins, the pterygoid and orbital plexus at the base of the brain. Ordinarily, transient obstruction of these collateral channels has no effect on venous outflow because more blood is channeled to the internal jugular. In intracranial hypertension, when elastance is high, these collateral venous channels carry more blood than usual.[27] Large increases in ICP can thus occur with obstruction of these plexus or the internal jugular vein. Both are obstructed by such activity as turning the head 90°.[27,28,29]

Venous outflow can further be obstructed by raising intrathoracic and intraabdominal pressure. Since the venous system has no valves, an increase in pressure will be transmitted to all portions. Those elevated intrathoracic pressures that would be of no consequence in health, become sources of increased ICP in the patient with high elastance. Examples of patient and critical care activities that increase intrathoracic and intraabdominal pressure include Valsalva's maneuver (breath holding, straining), positive end expiratory pressure, coughing and vomiting.

Increase in Cerebrospinal Fluid Volume. As discussed earlier, an increase in CSF through enhanced formation or decreased reabsorption can be a primary cause of intracranial hypertension. In the patient with existing intracranial hypertension, displacement of CSF caudad into the spinal cavity has already occurred to the extent that is possible. Any event that serves to retain even small "extra" amounts of CSF in the cranial cavity will act to increase ICP. Head rotation, flexion and extension, and perhaps even lying supine with a small pillow are examples of such situations. In a brain that is in a state of high elastance, such head movements can transiently obstruct the basal cisterns, interrupting free flow of CSF to the spinal cavity. It is likely that in such situations obstruction of venous and CSF outflow interact to create increases in ICP. Shalit and Umansky[30] measured ICP and jugular venous pressure simultaneously while rotating a patient's head 90°. Both pressures rose simultaneously, suggesting that obstruction of CSF channels led to the rise in both pressures, not that the jugular obstruction led to the ICP rise.

Summary

In the patient with intracranial hypertension, mechanisms that compensate for changes in any one of the three intracranial volumes have been exhausted. When ICP is thus increased, even very small changes in any of the three volumes can lead to large changes in pressure. A patient in this situation is said to be in a state of high elastance (or low compliance)—he or she has a "tight" brain. In such a state, situations that serve to increase blood pressure, cause cerebral vasodilatation, obstruct venous outflow, or obstruct spinal flow of CSF can create large transient or sustained increases over the already increased baseline ICP.

ASSESSMENT OF INTRACRANIAL HYPERTENSION

Direct measurement of intracranial pressure is the only clinically reliable and valid way to detect intracranial hypertension. Clinical signs and symptoms are not reliable in 1) detecting early intracranial hypertension; 2) determining the severity of increased ICP; or 3) determining if ICP is even elevated.[16,31–33]

The "classic" signs of increasing ICP (change in level of consciousness, change in pupil equality and reactivity, widening pulse pressure and bradycardia) are actually signs of brainstem dysfunction. If they occur in patients with intra-cranial hypertension, they indicate that neurologic status is worsening and that the brainstem is becoming compromised. If they occur in persons with normal ICP, they indicate primary brainstem damage. Prior to the advent of continuous ICP monitoring, these signs were correlated with increased ICP because the injuries that so often lead to brain herniation and brainstem dysfunction also often create intracranial hypertension related to expansion of brain volume or distortion of CSF pathways. With ICP monitoring, it is now evident that a number of patients with head injuries may have normal ICP but have signs of brainstem dysfunction,[32] that high levels of ICP may occur with relatively few symptoms,[14] and that a periodically deteriorating clinical condition may reflect very large increases in ICP superimposed on relatively asymptomatic baselines of elevated ICP.[16]

The foregoing is not to say that one relies on ICP monitoring alone and does not look at the patient. The observation of the patient's clinical status is crucial in detecting deterioration of his or her *neurologic* state, particularly the function of the brainstem.

To adequately evaluate the patient with intracranial hypertension, one must take into account these sets of data: intracranial pressure, cerebral per-fusion pressure, intracranial volume-pressure relationships, and clinical status.

Measuring Intracranial Pressure

Intracranial pressure may be measured continuously via the lateral ven-tricle or the subdural, epidural, or subarachnoid spaces (Fig. 2-2). For B and C, the pressure sensing device is connected by fluid-filled, pressure-resistant tubing to a transducer, which in turn is connected to a digital monitor and/or paper recorder.

Continuous measurement is preferable to the older single measurement of lumbar CSF pressure for two reasons. First, normal and abnormal variations in pressure are missed in single measurements. Secondly, the lumbar CSF pressure accurately reflects intracranial pressure only when lumbar and cranial CSF pathways communicate freely. Neural trauma and disease frequently dis-tort brain tissues and partially obstruct these channels, as do the ordinary activities of head turning and neck flexion discussed earlier. Additionally, when intracranial volumes are increased and compensated for only by displacement of CSF into the spinal cavity, withdrawal of such fluid for lumbar puncture creates a sudden pressure difference between cranial and spinal cavity and can cause herniation of the brain through the foramen magnum.[2]

Equipment for continuous monitoring is calibrated in either mm Hg (torr) or mm H_2O. It is preferable to use mm Hg to facilitate calculation of cerebral perfusion pressure, as discussed later.

The use of an intraventricular cannula is the most reliable and accurate means of monitoring ICP. Furthermore, this method allows withdrawal of CSF

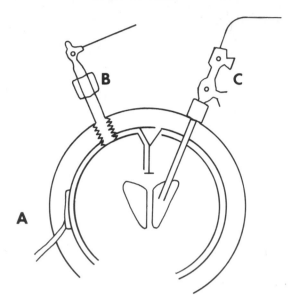

Fig. 2-2. Three methods of monitoring intracranial pressure. A is an epidural transducer, placed against the dura. B is a subarachnoid bolt, threaded into the skull and contacting the subarachnoid space. C is the intraventricular cannula, traversing both skull and brain tissue to reach a lateral cerebral ventricle.

to control pressure. Intraventricular cannulation is difficult when ventricles are small, as in grossly edematous brains, and there is always a small risk of infection, hemorrhage, and functional damage involved in traversing brain tissue.

Subdural, epidural, and subarachnoid devices do not enter brain tissue itself, but transform pulsations of the meninges into ICP measurements. There is still some risk of infection with these devices, as with intraventricular cannulas, as they are in contact with the meninges. They do not require invasion of brain tissue itself, and for this reason are preferred by many neurosurgeons. Swelling of brain tissue can occlude the measuring site in these sensors and result in damped and falsely low readings. Conversely, the meningeal sensors may be the only feasible device in brain swelling that results in ventricles too small to cannulate easily. The ICP values given by all the devices are correlated linearly (e.g., they all increase or decrease together), but the absolute magnitude is not equal. Epidural monitors in particular tend to give both higher and lower readings than do intraventricular methods.[34]

Cerebral Perfusion Pressure

The ICP level by itself is not a sufficient indicator of potential neuronal damage. In the critically ill patient, it is equally important to know the relationship between systemic blood pressure and ICP—the perfusion pressure.

Cerebral perfusion pressure (CPP) is defined as the difference between mean ICP and mean systemic arterial blood pressure (SABP). It is the effective pressure at which the brain cells are being perfused.

Sophisticated monitors can be programmed to display CPP provided both ICP and SABP are being monitored. If blood pressure is being estimated by auscultation, or if only systolic/diastolic data are displayed on the monitor, the following formulas may be used to calculate perfusion pressure. Both ICP and arterial blood pressure have systolic and diastolic points. Mean pressure for each can be calculated as follows:

$$\text{Mean ICP} = \text{diastolic ICP} + \tfrac{1}{3}\,\text{pulse pressure}$$

$$\text{where pulse pressure} = \text{systolic ICP} - \text{diastolic ICP}$$

Mean blood pressure is calculated substituting systolic and diastolic BP for ICP. Mean ICP is subtracted from mean BP to estimate CPP:

$$\text{CPP} = \text{mean BP} - \text{mean ICP}$$

Volume-Pressure Relationships

As described earlier, neither the ICP nor CPP alone can predict the likelihood in any given individual of large changes in ICP with small additions of volume. These values do not tell us where the patient is on the ICP volume/pressure curve. Such information can be derived clinically by use of the volume-pressure response (VPR) test of Miller,[10] or the pressure-volume index (PVI) of Marmarou.[11] Both can be calculated clinically by noting the change in ICP in response to a given volume added to the intracranial space.

The VPR is defined as ratio of immediate ICP response to a given volume of saline injected over 1 second. For example, if 1 ml saline is injected in 1 second and the ICP rises 1 torr, the VPR is 1 (1 torr/1 mm saline); if the ICP rises 2 torr, the VPR is 2. When it is too risky to inject 1 ml into the ventricle, smaller volumes can be used, with the ratio calculated accordingly. For example, 0.5 ml injected with 2 torr rise in ICP would yield a VPR of 4 (2 torr/.5 ml saline). Any VPR greater than 2 is significant.[10]

The PVI is based on the same principle but expresses the amount of volume that must be added to produce a tenfold increase in ICP. Since such large volumes would not actually be injected into patients at risk, the index can be estimated by recording a baseline pressure (P_0); injecting a bolus of a given volume (dV), and recording the peak pressure following injection (P_p). PVI is calculated as follows:

$$\text{PVI} = \frac{dV}{\log P_p / P_0}$$

In other words, the change in volume is divi᠁ ᠁ by the logarithm of the ratio of the peak pressure after injection to the baseline pressure. Thus, if the baseline ICP was 20 torr, 0.5 ml saline was injected and the peak pressure after injection was 40 torr, PVI would be as follows:

$$PVI = \frac{0.5}{0.301} \quad (\log 40/20 = \log 2 = 0.301)$$

$$PVI = 1.67$$

The PVI value means that only 1.67 ml of fluid would be required to raise ICP by a factor of 10. Such a low value indicates that the brain is very "tight," i.e., high in elastance. Normal PVI for an adult is approximately 25 ml.

Nonvolumetric Estimates of Elastance.   Obviously, use of the VPR or VPI poses some risk to the patient, since volume must be deliberately injected into the cranial cavity. Consequently, these quantitative measures are usually made by the neurosurgeon. In addition, very small volumes are used to challenge patients suspected of being in states of high elastance, and in pediatric patients who have much smaller total CSF volumes. Qualitative estimates of elastance can be made by noting the ICP response to such care activities as turning, suctioning, and spontaneous coughing.[4,35]

The amplitude and waveform of the ICP pulse wave can also provide qualitative evidence of decreasing compliance. The amplitude of the ICP trace is low in normal pressure states, but becomes increasingly wide as pressure and elastance increases. In addition, the cardiac pulse waveform can be distinguished from respiratory waves at higher ICP. Portnoy and colleagues have noted a change in waveform from sharp upswing to a more rounded form as compliance decreases and prior to any actual changes in ICP.[36] Such changes in waveform characteristics require relatively rapid paper speed to detect, however, many new monitors can be programmed to detect such changes through a technique known as spectral analysis.[36,37]

Clinical Neurologic Status

Although clinical signs are not good measures of levels and trends in ICP, they are crucial in detecting deteriorating neurologic status. Decreasing level of consciousness, focal motor weakness, abnormal posturing, inequality of pupils, loss of oculocephalic reflexes ("doll's eye" reflex), and changes in vital signs are clear indications of progressive brainstem dysfunction and brain herniation. Changes in brainstem reflexes are the only indicators of further deterioration in the unconscious patient. Consequently, it is important to periodically evaluate level of consciousness, motor function, ocular motility, respiratory patterns, and vital signs.

TREATMENT OF INTRACRANIAL HYPERTENSION

Intracranial hypertension is a symptom of disordered cranial volume-pressure relationships. Therefore, the primary aim of medical therapy is to diagnose and treat the *cause* of the increased ICP rather than merely treat the symptom.

Different modes of treatment affect different intracranial compartments. Thus, it becomes important to the physician to determine the cause of increased ICP in order to use the most rational therapy. In many cases, however, the ICP is sufficiently elevated to pose threat to survival of neurons if it is not reduced rapidly. In such cases, medical therapy may initially be aimed at reducing pressure by whatever means are available, while the physician is attempting simultaneously to determine and treat the primary cause.

The therapeutic aims of nursing in intensive care are twofold: 1) to support and implement the physician's therapy, and 2) to prevent environmentally induced rises in ICP, as far as possible. ICP monitoring enables both physician and nurse to see the effects of medical and nursing therapy, and to revise protocols, as necessary, for the individual patient.

Medical Therapies

Medical therapies are intended to reduce volume in the brain compartment that has expanded. Therapies may be surgical or medical. Surgical treatment may include removal of tumor; subdural, epidural, or intracerebral blood clot; or surgical decompression (removal of a piece of skull). Nonsurgical treatment is indicated in diffuse cerebral edema or to "buy time" to prepare for surgery.

Indications for Medical Therapy of Intracranial Hypertension. Elevation of ICP above 15–20 torr does not automatically mean that the physician will institute treatment to reduce it. Such a decision depends on the clinical state of the patient, the characteristics and trends of the recording, and the effect of the ICP on perfusion pressure. Most clinicians use guidelines similar to those of Bruce[4] and treat patients with continually rising baseline ICP once it reaches 20–25 torr; treat patients with pressure waves (periodic increases above an already increased baseline) that occur more often than once an hour and exceed 20–25 torr, or single pressure waves exceeding 30 torr. Goals of therapy include maintaining adequate cerebral blood flow, abolishing waves of pressure, preserving autoregulation (known to be lost in animals when ICP reaches about 30 torr) and reducing intracranial elastance.

General Therapy. In most institutions, patients who are being monitored either to detect intracranial hypertension or to follow the course of existing intracranial hypertension, require general supportive medical therapy to follow and treat both the systemic effects of the pathology and of the therapies for increased ICP. Patients with multiple trauma are particularly at risk for systemic problems that compound intracranial effects of trauma.[38] Adequate ventilation is crucial to prevent both hypoxia and hypercarbia. Assisted ventilation may be necessary in the unconscious patient to maintain PaO_2 80–100 torr. Hyperventilation to $PaCO_2$ of 25–30 torr is commonly used to keep intracranial vessels constricted and thereby reduce ICP without causing anaerobic metabolism.[18]

Systemic blood pressure must be supported to maintain cerebral blood flow. Any coexistent anemia, shock, or hypoproteinemia is treated to maintain systemic volume. Systemic hypertension may be treated carefully with antihypertensives, but requires continuous monitoring of both ICP and SABP to ensure adequate cerebral perfusion pressure.

Electrolytes and serum osmolality are monitored frequently. Although there are reports of inappropriate secretion of antidiuretic hormone (ADH) following head injury, excessive fluid replacement with nonosmotic intravenous fluids appears to contribute to the development of hypoosmolality in such patients.[39] Dextrose in water is a nonosmotic solution that should be avoided in neurosurgical patients. In addition, electrolytes and serum osmolality must be monitored closely when patients are receiving osmotic diuretics and loop diuretics.

Specific Medical Therapies.   *Hyperosmolar Agents.*   Drugs such as mannitol, urea, and glycerol act to draw fluid out of swollen brain cells by increasing the osmolarity of the blood. An intact blood-brain barrier (i.e., the tight junctions remain tight) is necessary in order that the large molecules of these agents do not diffuse into the brain and actually increase edema. Thus, these probably act to decrease normal interstitial water rather than to correct the pathophysiology underlying the edema.

Mannitol 20% has the least incidence of a rebound swelling (caused by slow diffusion of the molecules into the brain) and is the most commonly used. Usual dose is 0.5 to 1.5 gm/kg, given as a bolus. Serum osmolality must be comonitored and maintained at less than 315–320 mOsmol. Levels greater than this are associated with renal failure, seizures, further neurologic deterioration, and death. Mannitol acts rapidly (5–15 minutes) and maintains effect for several hours.

Furosemide and other diuretics have also been used effectively to reduce cerebral edema, perhaps by a combination of reduction of general body water and a direct effect on swollen glial cells. Glycerol and acetazolamide have been used in long-term disorders such as benign intracranial hypertension.[40]

Glucocorticoids.   The glucocorticoids have been accepted as effective in reducing edema associated with tumors. They have been used widely following stroke and head injury, but their efficacy has not been well documented in these situations. Support for high-dose dexamethasone grew after a German double-blind study;[41] however, the difference in outcome between the high-dose and low-dose groups was not statistically significant. Recent prospective double-blind studies that compared placebo, low-dose steroids, and high-dose steroids have not shown any difference in patient outcome in terms of ICP level or long-term outcome.[42–44] Long-term outcome indicators were non-specific or general in all studies (dead, vegetative existence, some recovery, good recovery) and do not measure well the quality of neurologic outcome.

Although steroids are often implicated in gastrointestinal bleeding in patients with head trauma, two recent studies have not found an increased incidence of gastrointestinal bleeding, hyperglycemia, or infection among patients treated with steroids versus those treated with placebo.[43,45] In summary, steroids in high doses do not appear to pose additional risks to patients with increased ICP following head injury, although the efficacy remains to be demonstrated.

Barbiturate Therapy. Coma induced by long- or short-acting barbiturates is increasingly used as therapy. The mechanism of the protective effect of barbiturates on brain function is not clear. Decrease in metabolic requirements, decrease in cerebral blood flow, and abolition of response to environmental stimuli are some of the mechanisms postulated.[46] Barbiturate coma in children with Reye's syndrome who have uncontrollable ICP has been reported to produce remarkable increase in survival.[47]

Barbiturate coma requires complete supportive care of a comatose, mechanically ventilated patient. Systemic effects on cardiac output and blood pressure require monitoring of SABP, pulmonary wedge pressure, and often, cardiac output. Blood pressure may drop sufficiently to compromise perfusion pressure, and dopamine may be given as indicated to restore SABP. The patient is not only comatose, but often without reflexes that protect airway, cornea, and skin. A management plan that combines nursing and medical therapy of such patients is reproduced in Table 2-1.[48]

Drainage of CSF. This therapy may be used when communicating or noncommunicating hydrocephalus complicates or is the main cause of the increased ICP. Fluid may be drained intermittently to bring pressure to predetermined levels, or continuously against positive pressure. The latter is preferred by many neurosurgeons to prevent rapid decompression of the ventricular system, and subsequent ventricular collapse and subdural hematoma as the brain pulls away from bridging vessels. Continuous or intermittent drainage requires ventriculostomy and direct penetration of the brain. Consequently, careful asepsis is necessary while maintaining a closed sterile system in all parts of the drainage apparatus.

Additional Therapies. Hypothermia is often used, particularly in children, to reduce metabolism and thereby demand for cerebral blood flow, cerebral blood volume, and ICP. Monitoring of cardiac rhythm and blood pressure are necessary because hypothermia depresses myocardial function and blood pressure, secondary to reduction of stroke volume. Cardiac arrhythmias and pulmonary edema are potential problems during rewarming when myocardial depression is reversed. Barbiturate therapy and hypothermia may be used in combination, and require careful monitoring of physiologic function, blood volume, and fluid balance.

Pancuronium (Pavulon) and morphine sulfate are often used as adjuncts to therapy to decrease the skeletal muscle and central response to environmental stimuli such as moving, turning, suctioning. Pancuronium may abolish the ICP waves secondary to tonic muscle contractions in patients who have abnormal motor posturing.

NURSING THERAPY

The critical care nurse has primary responsibility for preventing environmental stimuli that further increase ICP, in addition to exercising considerable judgment in implementing the medical protocols. A number of activities that

Table 2-1. Management of Patients in Induced Barbiturate Coma

Problem	Outcome	Management
Uncontrolled increased intracranial pressure (ICP > 20 torr for > 30 min and unresponsive to usual Rx methods)	ICP maintained at/less than 15 torr Cerebral perfusion pressure at least 60–70 mm Hg Temperature between 37°C to 38°C rectally	Monitor intracranial pressure continuously Calculate CCP (mean arterial pressure — ICP) qlh; notify physician if 50 mm Hg or less Fluid restriction of 80 cc/hr or as ordered Administer diuretics, e.g., mannitol, furosemide (Lasix[R]) as ordered Maintain normothermia with hypothermia-hyperthermia blanket and/or antipyretic agents
Adequate barbiturate level to control ICP	Serum barbiturate level maintained at about 3.0 mg% ICP at/less than 15 torr	Administer pentobarbital glh slowly intravenously as ordered (rate 10 min/100 mgm) Daily serum barbiturate levels
Hypotension due to cardiovascular instability and hypovolemia	Arterial systolic pressure maintained above 90 mm Hg Urinary output at least 30 cc/hr CVP and PAP within normal limits Normal sinus rhythm	Continuing monitoring of: Arterial pressure Pulmonary artery pressure Central venous pressure ECG pattern Check cuff pressure q shift and prn Administer vasopressor, e.g., dopamine if systolic < 90 mm Hg. (one dose of pentobarbital may be held) Urinary output qlh
Respiratory depression (unable to breath spontaneously, absence of cough reflex)	Arterial blood gases—PCO_2-within normal limits or 22–25 torr PO_2-100 torr Normal breath sounds bilaterally	Maintain on ventilator at 10–14/min and Sigh 10:2 ratio or as ordered Endotracheal tube or tracheostomy care Monitor cuff pressure continuously Suction and bag qlh and prn Irrigate tube with normal saline prn Suction nasopharyngeal secretions q2h and prn Arterial blood gases daily and prn Check breath sounds q 1–2h
Fluid and electrolyte imbalance 2° to fluid restrictions, diuretics, and GI suction	Serum osmolality < 320 mOsm Serum electrolytes within normal limits, e.g., Na, K Normal sinus rhythm Absence of T wave depression and U waves BUN, creatinine, and hematocrit within normal limits	Serum osmolality BID (hold mannitol, Lasix if > 320 mOsm and notify physician) Electrolytes, BUN, creatinine, Hct daily and prn Monitor PAP and ECG pattern continuously Urinary output and specific gravity qlh Total intake and output q24h and

Table 2-1. (*continued*)

Problem	Outcome	Management
	Absence of clinical signs of dehydration	cumulatively Observe skin and mucous membranes for evidence of dehydration
Gastrointestinal depression (absence of bowel sounds, inability to assimilate)	Absence of vomiting Absence of impaction Absorption of tube feedings	Salem-sump or nasogastric tube to gravity drainage or intermittent suction Measure gastric output q shift Auscultate for bowel sounds q shift and prn Palpate abdomen for distention Check for impaction Check gastric contents for assimilation when tube feedings are initiated after bowel sounds have returned
Loss of gag, swallow, and corneal reflexes	Absence of aspiration Absence of trauma to cornea	Suction oropharynx qh and prn Position on each side, avoid placing on back as much possible Cleanse eyes and apply liquid tears or Lacri-Lube^R q4h and prn Tape eyelids closed prn
Susceptibility to infection	WBC within normal limits Cultures negative	Strict aseptic technique Culture questionable sites prn
Inadequate nutrition due to catabolic state	Minimal weight loss	Multivitamins daily as ordered Parenteral hyperalimentation as ordered
Immobility	Absence of atelectasis Absence of skin breakdown Absence of thrombophlebitis and pulmonary embolism Absence of contractures	Institute appropriate preventive measures (specific details of care are beyond the scope of this paper)
Inability to cope and lack of understanding by the family/significant others	Verbalize realistic expectations Verbalize an appropriate understanding of the patient's condition and the therapy	Allow the family members to ventilate and ask questions Ask questions Give appropriate information without generating unrealistic expectations

Used by permission, from Ricci, M: Intracranial hypertension: barbiturate therapy and the role of the nurse. J Neurosurg Nurs 11:251–252, 1979.

are part of caring for the bedfast patient have been noted to increase ICP. These include turning the patient,[30,35,49] flexion, extension and rotation of the head,[27,30,49,50] suctioning,[26,30,35] PEEP,[51–53] positioning the patient prone,[50] emotionally disturbing conversion,[35] and combining several activities in succession.[35,49] Activities initiated by the patient such as use of the bedpan,[35,54] straining during elimination,[54,55] chewing,[35] coughing,[35,56,57] REM sleep,[35,55,58,59] periodic breathing,[16] and restlessness,[4,16,26] have also been associated with transient and sustained increases in ICP.

When ICP has increased subsequent to repositioning the patient, adjusting the position (e.g., through change of head position or change from supine to lateral) may reduce ICP.[30,49,50]

Not all patients experience increased ICP with these activities. It is likely that patients who do show these increases have high elastance and respond to small changes in intracranial volume induced by these activities; however, this has not been demonstrated experimentally. Mechanisms proposed to explain the effects of these stimuli include obstruction of venous outflow via the Valsalva maneuver, increased intrathoracic pressure and obstruction of the internal jugular vein,[26–29] obstruction of CSF basal cisterns,[30] increased regional CBF (emotion and REM sleep),[16,59] and vascular pressure waves secondary to rapid movement.[60]

Therefore, it can be proposed that patients with high VPR or PVI are at risk for ICP pressure peaks and pressure waves (5 minutes or greater increase beyond already elevated baseline). If the nurse does not have access to such quantitative estimates of intracranial elastance, indicators such as increased amplitude of ICP tracing, change in shape of ICP waveform (provided the recording system is patent), or ICP response to a given activity may roughly predict patients who may be in states of high elastance. While it cannot be predicted that a given activity will lead to increased ICP in a group of patients, investigators note consistency in response of individual patients to nursing care maneuvers.[4,26,49]

Patients whose ICP is uncontrollable by conventional means and whose ICP increases even further with a variety of nursing care and environmental stimuli, are increasingly treated with drugs that paralyze skeletal muscles (such as pancuronium chloride) or depress total central nervous system response (such as barbiturates or morphine sulfate). Such pharmocologic measures may reduce ICP response to nursing care and environmental stimuli. As discussed earlier, they are not benign drugs and require intensive monitoring and management of their effects on multiple body systems.

There are no published systematic studies that describe the effect on ICP of modifying the sequencing of nursing care activity or the manner of performing a specific maneuver. However, there is ample anecdotal documentation that ICP peaks induced by head rotation and neck flexion or extension can be reduced by restoring normal anatomic position. Lowering the patient's head to flat can raise ICP. While the usual position for patients with increased ICP is 15°–30°, it is not uncommon that patients who undergo multiple invasive monitoring are placed flat for measurement of such variables as central venous pressure or pulmonary wedge pressure. Such a practice is unnecessary provided that the measuring device remains at the phlebostatic level relative to the degree of head elevation.[61–64]

The prone position is not likely to be used in the critically ill patient, but should be avoided altogether in any patient with increased ICP.

In the absence of systematic intervention data, guidelines for nursing man-

Table 2-2. Mechanisms by which Patient Activities Increase ICP

Mechanism	Activity or Condition	Nursing Intervention
Increase in cerebral blood volume secondary to:		
1. Rise in blood pressure		
A. Isometric muscle contraction	Turning, moving up and down in bed, pushing self Decerebrate/decorticate posturing	Turning sheet, encourage awake patient to allow passive movement Avoid stimuli that cause posturing, if possible; phenothiazines, pancuronium may help
B. Rebound phase of Valsalva maneuver	Straining at stool	Prevent constipation; use stool softeners, suppositories as dictated by state of consciousness
	Pushing self, moving in bed	Encourage patient to exhale while turning, pushing up in bed
C. Emotional stimuli	Family visits, conversation about fears, concerns	Weigh risks vs. benefit for each person; avoid conversations held "over" patient about condition
2. Decreased venous outflow		
A. Transient mechanical obstruction to jugular, vertebral, and intrathoracic venous systems	Head and body position that obstructs flow: rotated head; flexed, extended neck; extreme hip flexion	Keep head in neutral position when possible, avoid neck flexion and extension both in resting posture and during procedures Slight head up position promotes venous drainage
B. Increased intrathoracic and intraabdominal pressure	Any activity that causes a Valsalva maneuver Body positions that increase pressure: prone, extreme hip flexion	See previous intervention re: Valsalva
	Positive end-expiratory pressure ventilation (PEEP) in some patients	Head up position may help; avoid multiple activities in patients who increase ICP with PEEP
3. Cerebral vasodilatation secondary to hypercapnia or marked hypoxia (PaO_2) 50–60 torr	Occluded airway	Keep airway patent; if suctioning necessary, use intermittent, brief (15 s or less) periods; may help to preoxygenate the patient
Increase in CSF volume Transient increase in intracranial CFS due to obstruction of basal cisterns	Head position that temporarily occludes CFS outflow to spinal sac: head rotation, neck extension	Avoid head rotation whenever possible; side-lying position may be helpful to patients with decreased CFS absorption (such as post subarachnoid hemorrhage)

[a] From Mitchell, P: AACN Clinical Reference for Critical Care Nursing. Chapter 26. In M. Kinney et al, Eds. McGraw Hill, New York, 1980.

agement can be inferred from the available data regarding the effects of various activity on ICP (Table 2-2). Patients with increased ICP should be kept in a 15°–30° head elevated position, even when transported. The head should remain in good alignment in all body positions; extreme rotation, flexion, and extension should be avoided. If ICP rises consistently when the patient is turned to any given position, that position should be avoided if possible. If turning induces ICP increase, conscious patients can be instructed to let the nurse turn them passively to avoid the effects on blood pressure of isometric muscle contraction and Valsalva maneuver.

If ICP increases in a patient following a given care activity, it is likely to continue to do so when that activity is repeated. If the care activity can be avoided, so much the better. If it cannot, the nurse may use the ICP readings to gauge the effect of any modification in care. Such activity may have a lesser effect on ICP if it does not closely follow other care activities, particularly those known to increase ICP. It may be helpful to turn patients more slowly or use mechanical rotating beds, such as Rotorest.

Short suctioning periods (10–15 seconds) may be as important in preventing hypoxia-induced elevations in ICP as any hyperoxygenation or hyperventilation prior to suctioning. Good bowel programs started early can prevent the hard, impacted stools that result in straining, even in unconscious patients. Finally, management of the environment can include avoiding loud, sudden noises, abrupt bumping of the bed, and emotionally disturbing conversation within earshot of both conscious and unconscious patients.

While much research is needed to identify efficacious nursing interventions in groups of patients with ICP elevations, each critical care nurse can use ICP monitoring and clinical status assessment to determine therapeutic and harmful nursing activity in any given patient.

REFERENCES

1. Langfitt TW: Increased intracranial pressure. Clin Neurosurg 16:436–471, 1969.
2. Plum F, Posner JB: The Diagnosis of Stupor and Coma. pp. 114–116. 3rd Ed. FA Davis, Philadelphia, 1980.
3. Miller, JD: Volume and pressure in the craniospinal axis. Clin Neurosurg 22:76–105, 1975.
4. Bruce DA: The pathophysiology of increased intracranial pressure. Upjohn Company, 1978.
5. Lofgren J, Zwetnow NN: Cranial and spinal components of the cerebrospinal fluid pressure volume curve. Acta Neurol Scand 49:575–585, 1973.
6. Davson H: Physiology of the Cerebrospinal Fluid. p. 4. Little-Brown Co., Boston, 1967.
7. Martins AN, Wiley JK, Myers PW: Dynamics of the cerebrospinal fluid and the spinal dura mater. J Neurol Neurosurg Psychiatr 35:468–473, 1972.
8. Miller JD, Leech P: Effects of mannitol and steroid therapy on intracranial volume-pressure relationships in patients. J Neurosurg 42:274–281, 1975.

9. Langfitt TW: Where have we been, where are we now, and where do we go from here? In Shulman, K, et al, Eds: Intracranial Pressure IV. pp. 669–676. Springer-Verlag, Berlin, 1980.

10. Miller JD, Garibi J: Intracranial volume/pressure relationship during continuous monitoring of ventricular fluid pressure. In Brock M, Dietz H, Eds: Intracranial Pressure. pp. 270–274. Springer-Verlag, Berlin, 1972.

11. Marmarou A, Shulman K, Rosende R: A non-linear analysis of the cerebrospinal fluid system and intracranial pressure dynamics. J Neurosurg 48:332–334, 1978.

12. Miller JD, Becker DP, Ward JD et al: Significance of intracranial hypertension in severe head injury. J Neurosurg 47:503–516, 1977.

13. Lassen NA: Control of the cerebral circulation in health and disease. Circ Res 34:746–760, 1974.

14. Johnston IH, Paterson, A: Benign intracranial hypertension. Brain 97:301–312, 1974.

15. Greenberg RP, Mayer DJ, Becker DP: Correlation in man of intracranial pressure and neuroelectric activity determined by multimodality evoked potentials. In Beks JWF, Ed: Intracranial Pressure III. pp. 58–62. Springer-Verlag, Berlin, 1976.

16. Lundberg N: Continuous recording and control of ventricular fluid pressure in neurosurgical practice. Acta Psych Neurol Scand 36(suppl) 149, 1960.

17. Fishman RA: Brain edema. N Eng J Med 293:700–711, 1975.

18. Miller JD: The management of cerebral oedema. Br J Hosp Med 21(2):152–166, 1979.

19. Ignelzi RJ: Cerebral edema: Present perspectives. Neurosurg 4:338–342, 1979.

20. Reivich M: Regulation of cerebral circulation. Clin Neurosurg 16:378, 1968.

21. Grubb RL, et al: The effects of changes in $PaCo_2$ on cerebral blood volume, blood flow, and vascular mean transit time. Stroke 5:630–639, 1974.

22. Borgstrom L, Johannsson H, Siesjo B: The relationship between arterial PO_2 and cerebral blood flow in hypoxic hypoxia. Acta Physiol Scand 93:423–432, 1975.

23. Cohen PJ, Alexander SC, Smith TC, et al: Effects of hypoxia and normocarbia on cerebral blood flow and metabolism in conscious man. J Appl Physiol 23:183–189, 1967.

24. Fell T, Cheney FW: Prevention of hypoxia during endotracheal suction. Ann Surg 174:24–28, 1971.

25. Naigow D, Powaser MM: The effect of different endotracheal suction procedures on arterial blood gases in a controlled experimental model. Heart and Lung 6:808–816, 1977.

26. Shapiro HM: Intracranial hypertension: Therapeutic and anesthetic considerations. Anesthesiology 43:445–467, 1976.

27. Hulme A, Cooper R: The effects of head position and jugular vein compression on intractanial pressure. In Beks J, et al, Ed: Intracranial Pressure III. pp. 259–263. Springer-Verlag, Berlin, 1976.

28. Lipe HP, Mitchell PH: Positioning the patient with intracranial hypertension: How turning and head rotation affect the internal jugular vein. Heart and Lung 9:1031–1077, 1980.

29. Watson GN: Effect of head rotation on jugular vein flow. Arch Dis Child 49:237–239, 1974.

30. Shalit MN, Umansky R: Effect of bedside procedures on intracranial pressure. Israel J Med Sci 13:881–886, 1977.

31. Guillaume J, Janny P: Manometric intracranienne continue. Interet de la methode et premiens resultats. Rev Neurol 84:131–142, 1951.

32. Johnston IH, Johnston JA, Jennet B: Intracranial pressure changes following head injury. Lancet 2:433–436, 1970.
33. Pathak SN, et al: Vital signs in progressive intracranial hypertension: An experimental study. Indian J Med Res 60:859–869, 1972.
34. Zierski J: Extradural, ventricular and subdural pressure recording: Comparative clinical study. In Shulman K, et al, Eds: Intracranial Pressure IV. pp. 371–376. Springer-Verlag, Berlin, 1980.
35. Mitchell PH, Mauss NK: Relationship of patient-nurse activity to intracranial pressure variations: A pilot study. Nurs Res 27:4–10, 1978.
36. Portnoy HD, Chopp M: Spectral analysis of intracranial pressure. In Shulman K, et al, Eds: Intracranial Pressure IV. pp. 167–172. Springer-Verlag, Berlin, 1980.
37 Szweczykowski J, et al: Spectral analysis of the ICP signal—practical application in computer-assisted long-term patient care. In Shulman K, et al, Eds: Intracranial Pressure IV. pp. 419–422. Springer-Verlag, Berlin, 1980.
38. Miller JD, Sweet RC, Narayan R, Becker DP: Early insults to the injured brain. JAMA 240:439–442, 1978.
39. Steinbok P, Thompson GB: Metabolic disturbances after head injury: Abnormalities of sodium and water balance with special reference to the effects of alcohol intoxication. Neurosurg 3:9–15, 1978.
40. Quest DO: Dehydrating agents commonly used in neurosurgery: Advantages and disadvantages. J Neurosurg Nurs 11:141–143, 1979.
41. Gobiet W, Bock WJ, Leisegang J, et al: Treatment of acute cerebral edema with high-dose dexamethasone. In Beks JWF, et al, Eds: Intracranial Pressure III. pp. 231–235. Springer-Verlag, Berlin, 1976.
42. Gudeman, SK, Miller JO, Becker DP: Failure of high-dose steroid therapy to influence intracranial pressure in patients with severe head injury. J Neurosurg 51:301–306, 1979.
43. Cooper PR, Moody S, Clark WK, Kirkpatrick J, Maravilla F, Gould AL, Drane W: Dexamethasone and severe head injury: A prospective double-blind study. J Neurosurg 51:307–316, 1979.
44. Pitts LA, Kaktis JV: Effect of megadose steroids on ICP in traumatic coma. In Shulman K, et al, Eds: Intracranial Pressure IV. pp. 638–642. Springer-Verlag, Berlin, 1980.
45. Kaktis J, Pitts LH: Complications associated with use of megadose corticosteroids in head-injured patients. J Neurosurg Nurs 12:166–171, 1980.
46. Marshall LF, Smith RW, Shapiro HM: The outcome with aggressive treatment in severe head injuries, part II: Acute and chronic barbiturate administration in the management of head injury. J Neurosurg 50:26–30, 1979.
47. Bruce DA, Raphaely RA, Swedlow D, Schut L: The effectiveness of barbiturate coma in controlling increased ICP in 61 children. In Shulman K, et al, Eds: Intracranial Pressure IV. pp. 630–632. Springer-Verlag, Berlin, 1980.
48. Ricci MM: Intracranial hypertension: Barbiturate therapy and the role of the nurse. J Neurosurg Nurs 11:247–252, 1979.
49. Mitchell PH, Mauss NK, Ozuna J, Lipe H: Moving the patient in bed: Effects on intracranial pressure. Nurs Res 30:212–218, 1981.
50. Nornes H, Magnaes B: Supratentorial epidural pressure recorded during posterior fossa surgery. J Neurosurg 35:541–549, 1971.
51. Apuzzo M, et al: Effect of PEEP on intracranial pressure in man. J Neurosurg 46:227–232, 1977.

52. Aidinis SJ, Lafferty L, Shapiro HM: Intracranial responses to PEEP. Anesthesiology 45:275–286, 1976.
53. Frost EAM: Effects of positive end-expiratory pressure on intracranial pressure and compliance in brain injured patients. J Neurosurg 47:195–200, 1978.
54. Yoneda S, et al: Continuous measurement of intracranial pressure with SFT: Clinical experiences. Surg Neurol 4:289–295, 1975.
55. Symon L, Dorsch NW: Use of long-term intracranial pressure measurement to assess hydrocephalic patients prior to shunt surgery. J Neurosurg 42:258–273, 1975.
56. Bedford RF, et al: Lidocaine prevents increased ICP after endotracheal intubation. In Shulman K, Ed: Intracranial Pressure IV. Springer-Verlag, Berlin, 1980.
57. Williams, B: Cerebrospinal fluid pressure changes in response to coughing. Brain 99:331–346, 1976.
58. Gucer G, Viernstein LJ: Intracranial pressure in the normal monkey while awake and asleep. J Neurosurg 51:206–210, 1979.
59. Hulme A, Cooper R: Cerebral blood flow during sleep in patients with raised intracranial pressure. Prog Brain Res 30:77–81, 1968.
60. Magnaes B: Body position and cerebrospinal fluid pressure, Part I: Clinical studies on the effect of rapid postural change. J Neurosurg 44:687–697, 1976.
61. Strong A: Effects of patient positioning on central venous pressure measurements. Circulation 52(4):Suppl II:264, 1975.
62. Woods S: Techniques for pulmonary artery pressure measurement. Final report, Division of Nursing DHHS, Wash., D.C., 1980.
63. Woods S, Mansfield LW: Effect of backrest position on pulmonary wedge pressure in non-acutely ill patients. Heart and Lung 5:83–97, 1976.
64. Grose BL, et al: Effect of backrest position on thermodilution cardiac output measurement in 30 acutely ill patients. Circulation 60(4)Suppl II:248, 1979.

3 | Cardiovascular Complications of Intracranial Disorders

Ellen McCarthy

To function most effectively, the nurse working with neurological and neurosurgical patients must have a thorough understanding of the nervous system and the manifestations of disorders of that system. The future nurse will function in an expanded role with expanded responsibilities, recognized as a fellow professional and an active part of the neurological/neurosurgical team.[1] In addition to performing a neurological examination, nurses need to be able to evaluate neurological signs and symptoms, recognize impending and existing complications, and, if necessary, initiate treatment based on protocols or standardized procedures. Nurses need to further utilize the opportunity they have from continuous contact with patients to make pertinent clinical observations and correlate signs and symptoms with neurological pathology. Verbal and written communications with other health team members will contribute to the accumulation of nursing and medical knowledge. With this in mind, this paper presents the complex subject of cardiovascular implications of intracranial disorders, hoping to stimulate the experienced critical care nurse to investigate this fascinating subject further.

It is recognized that many neurological disorders result from cardiac and/ or vascular problems. These include (1) cerebral emboli that originate in the heart from artificial heart valves, mitral stenosis, bacterial endocarditis, post-myocardial infarction mural thrombosis, atrial fibrillation or other intermittent cardiac dysrhythmias; (2) cerebral ischemia secondary to hemodynamic

53

changes from dysrhythmias or heart block, especially if accompanied by cerebral atherosclerosis[2,3]; (3) cerebral thrombosis as a manifestation of atherosclerotic cardiovascular disease; (4) cerebral hemorrhage from anomalies or injuries to the cerebral arteries; (5) encephalopathy or intracranial hemorrhage resulting from hypertension.

Conversely, cardiovascular (CV) changes and problems may occur secondary to neurological injury. Many of these CV events are still not well understood. Continuing research is attempting to decrease the controversies surrounding the etiology, extent, and treatment of alterations in cerebral blood flow and observed hemodynamic and electrocardiographic (ECG) changes that occur in the patient with central nervous system (CNS) insult.

To understand the postulated CV events and their implications following neurological disorders, one must first be familiar with normal control of the systemic and cerebral circulation. Although there are some similarities between the two, the cerebral circulation is believed to have special regulatory mechanisms. The reader unfamiliar with the nervous, humoral, and local control of systemic blood flow would do well to review them to better understand the changes that occur with intracranial disorders.

REGULATION OF CEREBRAL CIRCULATION

The normal cerebral blood flow of the average adult is approximately 55–60 ml/100 gm brain/min (900–1100 ml/min) or 15–20 percent of the total resting cardiac output.[4,5] Cerebral blood flow (CBF) continually provides the vital nutrients of glucose and oxygen to brain cells. Decreased CBF severely compromises brain functioning, as the cells have the ability to store only minimal amounts of glucose and oxygen. Changes in CBF also can adversely affect the chemical and physical environment of the brain.

CBF is influenced by cerebral perfusion pressure and the diameter of the cerebrovascular bed. Cerebral perfusion pressure can be easily calculated in the patient whose intracranial pressure (ICP) is being monitored, and it allows for the assessment of CBF. In individuals with normal ICP, the jugular venous pressure is sometimes used to approximate ICP. However, because the jugular vein is outside the cranium, it does not correspondingly rise with increases in ICP. In patients with a neurological insult, therefore, cerebral perfusion pressure (CPP) is the difference between mean arterial blood pressure (MAP) and mean intracranial pressure (ICP) measured directly.

$$CPP = MAP - ICP$$

Maintenance of adequate perfusion pressure is critically important to avoid brain ischemia. Normal CPP ranges about 80–90 torr. If there is either a rise in ICP or a decline in MAP, CPP will be decreased.

$$\downarrow MAP - \uparrow ICP = \downarrow CPP$$

Under normal circumstances the autonomic nervous system appears to have little influence on CBF. Though richly innervated by sympathetic fibers, stimulation of the sympathetic fibers causes only a mild vasoconstriction of the large cerebral vessels, while stimulation of the parasympathetic fibers causes a mild vasodilation. It has been proposed therefore that the sympathetic nervous system may be only a crude adjustor of CBF,[5] and that the diameter of the vascular bed is influenced by additional factors such as autoregulation, local metabolites, arterial blood gases, and cerebral blood volume.

Within mean arterial pressures of approximately 60 and 160 torr, cerebral blood flow is fairly constant and independent of perfusion pressure, a phenomenon known as autoregulation. Though the exact mechanism is unknown, autoregulation is thought to be an intrinsic mechanism whereby cerebrovascular arteries respond to changes in CPP by altering their diameter in order to maintain a relatively constant flow in the microcirculation over a range of pressures.[6] A recent study by MacKenzie et al[7] indicated that the smaller arterioles were more reactive and increased their caliber by a larger percentage (93%) than either larger arterioles or small arteries (56%). This was in contrast to other areas of the body where precapillary sphincters and arterioles are the primary site of vascular resistance.[7] In addition, they found that although autoregulation became inadequate and could no longer compensate for decreasing perfusion pressure below 65 torr, vessels were not yet maximally dilated, and vasodilatation continued until the arterial pressure fell to 30–39 torr.[7]

Various factors alter autoregulation. Chronic hypertension shifts the limits of autoregulation upwards.[8] Following cerebral injury, autoregulation may be impaired either globally or regionally. Impaired autoregulation results in the inability of vascular smooth muscle in injured areas of the brain to actively oppose changes in perfusion pressure, and CBF varies directly with changes in arterial blood pressure.

It is now generally recognized that various areas of the brain have differing functions and metabolic needs, with corresponding differences in regional cerebral blood flow (rCBF).[6,9] For example, nuclear structures or gray matter have blood flow rates three to four times that of white matter.[4,5] Although the total blood supply within the brain remains fairly constant, rapid redistribution of the blood can occur as metabolic needs change in different areas (a functional hyperemia). These physiological changes are thought to occur secondary to increased local concentrations of metabolites that are vasoactive and dilate terminal arterioles. However, in circumstances where there is a significant increase in activity over large areas of the brain, such as generalized seizures, a corresponding increase in overall CBF occurs. Generalized seizures have been shown to increase CBF as much as 50 percent.[6,10] In contrast, pathological states often depress brain function and are accompanied by reduced metabolic rates and CBF. Examples include barbiturate intoxication and metabolic encephalopathies. However, there are a few exceptions, such as in hypoxia and ketoacidosis, where CBF is increased in spite of a low metabolic rate, probably

edema and increased venous pressure or obstruction that usually accompanies increased ICP. A recent study by McGillicuddy[11] indicated that there is virtually no CBF in arterioles at ICP levels sufficient to initiate the hypertensive response. Although a rising systemic arterial pressure and bradycardia in a head-injured patient would signal the probability of increasing ICP, the clinical usefulness of Cushing's reaction is limited in that it is a very late sign of raised ICP and often does not occur even in the presence of documented increased ICP. Blood pressure does not change until ICP exceeds arterial pressure, wherein it rises until diastolic pressure exceeds ICP.[11] Recent research supports the fact that blood pressure and heart rate changes are not reliable indicators of increased ICP[17,18] and waiting for them to occur could be disastrous.[19] Jachuck reports that Cushing's reaction does not appear until ICP exceeds 45 torr and the patient begins to become obtunded. At lower levels of elevated ICP, patients tend to be restless and have tachycardias.[20] In McGillicuddy's study, bradycardia signaled impending cardiovascular decompensation and was most commonly associated with concomitant hypoxia.[11] Cushing's reaction, therefore, is probably more of a "cry of distress" rather than a means of rescue for the injured brain.[15]

There is evidence to suggest that the rate of ICP rise may make a difference in the clinical response of the patient. If ICP rises slowly, arterial pressure also slowly increases to a level approximately 10 mm above intracranial pressure.[21] Occasionally, a periodic rise and fall in blood pressure above and below the level of increased intracranial pressure occurs. These fluctuations are called Traube-Hering waves and are probably due to a continuous feedback system. In contrast, a sharp rise in BP accompanies an abrupt increase in ICP[15] and has been shown to cause cardiac standstill of 10–20 seconds duration, apnea and incontinence. This is believed to be mediated through the vagus nerve (probably a vagovagal reflex) since experimentally, this response can be eliminated by vagotomy.[21] Following this initial response, there usually is a resumption of cardiac activity with tachycardia and increased arterial pressure, and the resumption of respirations.

Marshall[18] suggested a pattern of increased intracranial pressure during the early morning hours (4–9 a.m.) may be due to an increase in brain blood volume directly related to diurnal biorhythms. This may account for the decompensation of some brain-injured patients that occurs during sleep. It is postulated that treatment of these patients with IV barbiturates results in cerebral vasoconstriction with subsequent reduction of cerebral blood volume. This implies that raised intracranial pressure in head injury may sometimes be due to cerebrovascular causes rather than to brain edema solely related to the injury. In addition, there may be implications for more attention to cyclical biological activity, including CV changes, in selecting treatment for such patients.[15,18] Consideration of biological rhythms has long been the concern of many nurses in planning patient interventions. Because of the continual observations of patients, nurses have a unique opportunity to further identify and document this and possibly other diurnal rhythms present in the neurological patient that may influence the response to various treatments.

Cerebral Ischemia

Insufficient CBF to the brain indicates ischemia whether or not there is adequate oxygenation. It may be either diffuse, as is seen with cardiopulmonary arrest, or focal, as seen in stroke. It appears that ischemia can produce a greater risk of irreversible brain damage than profound hypoxia alone, since the toxic metabolic products (i.e., lactic acid) are not removed.[4] At a critical level of decreased CBF, not yet specifically identified in man, the electrical potential fails resulting in electroencephalograph (EEG) slowing. Potassium leaks from cells and the high extracellular concentrations can cause seizures.[4] Autoregulation is impaired in ischemic tissue and therefore changes in perfusion pressure will be reflected to the capillary bed, and even moderate hypertension can lead to increased cerebral edema; hypotension results in decreased CBF, contributing further to ischemia. Attention to moderate alterations in blood pressure then becomes extremely important to the nurse caring for patients with cerebral ischemia.

With the loss of autoregulation, the resting vasoconstrictor tone may be normal even though the vessels no longer have the ability to dilate or constrict. As ischemia progresses, there is a loss of this resting tone and the vessels become dilated in their resting state (termed *vasomotor paralysis*).[22] In focal ischemia, an apparent paradoxical situation has been identified in which there appears to be an initial preservation of autoregulation in severely injured tissue. However, more recently it has been hypothesized that this is due to increased tissue pressure from edema in the damaged areas rather than to active vasoconstriction.[23]

Vasomotor paralysis impairs responsiveness to changes in $PaCO_2$ in severe cerebral injury. For example, Enevoldsen and Jensen[23] reported impaired CO_2 vascular response in deeply comatose patients, which returned to normal as the patient recovered. Altered CO_2 response can result in an *intracerebral steal* or diversion of blood flow away from the ischemic area when the $PaCO_2$ is increased.[5,24] This is because vasomotor paralysis in the ischemic area does not allow vasodilatation to occur. The blood flow then shifts to the normal vascular bed, increasing the degree of ischemia in the injured area. Conversely, lowering the $PaCO_2$ may allow passive increased CBF to the ischemic area by causing vasoconstriction (only in reactive vessels[15]) and a shift of blood away from normal tissue. This is known as the *inverse steal phenomenon*.[6,24] Clinically, hyperventilation might be expected to increase blood flow to the ischemic area based on this inverse steal phenomenon.[24]

Ginsberg and Reivich[24] report various other treatment modalities for focal ischemia based on the problem of vasomotor paralysis. In addition to altering CO_2, the recommendations for restoring CBF have included the use of both vasodilator therapy and hypertensive therapy. Hypertensive therapy in stroke, though not well established or proven, is based on the rationale that autoregulation is lost in the ischemic area and elevation of blood pressure will therefore be passively transmitted to the ischemic region, increasing CBF. Vasodilators such as nitroprusside have been recommended in the hope that dilatation of the vessels supplying the ischemic area will increase flow. However, it is not known whether these vessels have the ability to dilate, or whether vasodilators merely contribute to the intracerebral steal phenomenon by dilating only vessels in normal tissue.

Another alteration of CBF that occurs with ischemia is *diaschisis.* Following an acute focal infarct, CBF may be decreased in the entire ipsilateral hemisphere and occasionally in the contralateral hemisphere. The exact mechanism of this action is still unknown, and therefore no specific recommendations for prevention or treatment have been proposed.[5,24] Ischemia also alters vascular permeability and the integrity of the blood-brain barrier causing vasogenic cerebral edema. External compression of the vascular bed by edematous tissue may further limit cerebral circulation. Recommendations for treating cerebral edema include hyperosmotic agents such as mannitol or glycerol. However, their effectiveness may require an intact blood-brain barrier, and there is evidence that repeated high doses of hyperosmolar agents result in leaking of the agent into the injured interstitial tissue. A reverse osmotic gradient is then established which draws fluid from the vasculature into the injured area leading to a "rebound" cerebral edema.[25] The use of steroids also has been recommended to decrease vasogenic edema. However, the effectiveness of steroids appears to be limited to chronic edematous states rather than acute injuries.[25,26]

Although under normal circumstances regional cerebral blood flow (r CBF) coincides with cerebral metabolism and function, this relationship does not exist in injured brain tissue. Studies have shown that there is reduced or absent rCBF in the center of an area of infarct, but hyperemia in the surrounding ischemic tissue.[5] This has been called a *luxury perfusion syndrome,* as there appears to be an uncoupling of metabolic needs and rCBF.[6,24] A possible cause is the accumulation of tissue lactic acidosis with vasodilatation in the still reactive perifocal vessels,[38] but this has not been proven. While rCBF measurements can now be done clinically, the lack of certainty about the relationship of rCBF to function in diverse states obscures the significance of abnormal measurements in the monitoring of various treatment modalities.[6] It should also be kept in mind that collateral circulation may develop if cerebral perfusion pressure is maintained, and thereby lead to variable functional deficits in different patients with occlusion of the same vessel.[5]

Global brain ischemia, resulting from cardiopulmonary arrest, hypotension, or increased ICP has been the subject of much recent research. *Brain resuscitation* is aimed at preservation of neurons following an episode of ischemia-anoxia. Safar pointed out that "for the next few decades, combinations of pharmacological and physiological measures are likely to evolve from various laboratories, being constantly modified and improved upon as they are taken to patients."[27] Extending the traditional ABCs (airway, breathing, and circulation) of basic life support and the DEFs (drugs and fluids, ECG, and fibrillation treatment) of advanced life support, Safar et al[28] have recently identified the importance of the GHIs (gauging the soundness of continuing resuscitative efforts, humanizing resuscitation with neuron-saving measures, and intensive care) of prolonged life support.

Global ischemia results in cytotoxic cerebral edema with paralysis of the sodium-potassium pump and autolysis. Even with the resumption of adequate CPP reperfusion after global ischemia is nonhomogeneous and there are frequently focal areas of impaired flow in the microvasculature.[29] This *no-reflow phenomenon* has been apparent after 5 to $7\frac{1}{2}$ minutes of cerebral circulatory arrest. Although the exact mechanism is unknown, capillary occlusion or compression secondary to cellular swelling, increased blood viscosity, and aggregation of erythrocytes have been implicated as causes of the no-reflow phenomenon.[5,24,28] The significance of this phenomenon as a factor in the location or extent of neurological deficit is as yet unproved. There is speculation that the situation may be improved with sufficiently high CPP.[29]

CO_2 response and autoregulation also are impaired in global ischemia. ICP remains near normal, however, unless there is extensive edema of cerebral tissue from prolonged and severe ischemia.[28] In severe shock, MAP below 30 torr for 15 min or more appears to be as injurious as cardiac arrest.[28] Maintenance of adequate arterial pressure and avoidance of hypertension are as important in global ischemia as they are in focal ischemia. Prevention and treatment of respiratory depression with resultant hypoxemia and hypercarbia is paramount. In addition, hemodilution to promote microcirculation, steroids to stabilize cell membranes and reduce edema, and osmotherapy to reduce cerebral edema have been tried. Barbiturate administration to the level of light anesthesia has been used as a means of suppressing metabolism at the neuronal level in the hope of protecting against ischemia and edema.[28] However, the effectiveness of this therapy remains controversial.

Fluctuations in Arterial Pressure

Arterial pressure fluctuations in brain injured patients also lead to variable CBF. Due to autoregulation, CBF is essentially independent of mean arterial blood pressure until pressure falls to about 50 percent of normal.[30] However, CBF will fall abruptly with possible resultant anoxic encephalopathy if CPP drops below 40 torr.[31] This may occur at mean arterial pressures as high as 80 torr if ICP is elevated to levels of 40 torr or more. Brain injured patients with increased ICP who experience only one episode of severe hypotension may develop perisulcal infarcts[32]—areas of necrosis in the deep cortical regions surrounding the cerebral sulci.

At the other extreme, if CPP rises 30 to 40 torr above normal values[9] or MAP is greater than 160 torr,[5] the limits of autoregulation are exceeded and CBF and ICP become passively related to blood pressure.[33] Loss of autoregulation and elevated arterial pressure therefore allow the hydrostatic pressure to be transmitted more directly to the capillaries. Overdistention of capillaries occurs and leads to a breakdown of the blood-brain barrier with leakage of plasma proteins into the interstitium. The osmotic gradient produced by the plasma proteins contributes to cerebral edema and further increased ICP and may lead to diminished CPP and CBF.

The goal of therapy for patients with impaired autoregulation is to maintain CPP without a significant elevation of arterial pressure,[6] since elevation of arterial pressure, in an effort to preserve CPP, is at the expense of transmission of high pressures to the capillary bed. In the presence of extremely elevated ICP, the ICP fluctuates with a change in arterial pressure. However, it is generally recommended to treat the cause of the elevated ICP rather than manipulate the blood pressure. In a patient with cerebral edema where CBF is already reduced, lowering blood pressure by artificial means may reduce CPP and CBF further.

Cerebral Arterial Spasm

Cerebral arterial spasm commonly develops in patients with a ruptured intracranial aneurysm or following local surgical trauma. It usually involves the arteries at the base of the brain,[4] and ICP remains near normal; however, it may occur days to weeks following rupture of an aneurysm. Vasospasm may result in cerebral ischemia and is associated with increased patient morbidity and mortality. The consequences of cerebral vasospasm include thrombosis and infarction distal to the constriction, leading to further nervous tissue damage. Clinically, the patient may begin to deteriorate with progressive unresponsiveness and neurologic deficit. Vasospasm may also occur following surgical repair of the aneurysm, and an incidence of 40 to 65 percent has been reported.[34] Currently it is thought that vasospasm results from the release of vasoactive substances such as serotonin, histamine, or prostaglandins. It has been postulated that the delay in onset of vasospasm is due to the time necessary for tissue breakdown and release of these substances.[24] Schmidek hypothesized that these substances are released from the blood into the cerebral spinal fluid (CSF) at the time of hemorrhage, but does not explain the delay.[34]

Treatment of cerebral vasospasm is still uncertain. Miller and Sullivan reported clinical improvement by inducing short-term arterial hypertension.[15] Allen reported the successful use of nitroprusside in the treatment of cerebral vasospasm following subarachnoid hemorrhage,[35] and nitroprusside has been used during neurosurgery to induce systemic hypotension to allow safer dissection of intracranial aneurysms and other vascular lesions.[36] Nitroprusside has a direct vasodilatory effect on systemic blood vessels, independent of the autonomic nervous system, and it is presumed to have similar effects on the cerebral vessels.[37] It has been reported that adequate CBF is maintained during the use of nitroprusside in spite of systemic hypotension[38] although some researchers advocate simultaneous administration of dopamine.[37] Apparently, moderate doses of dopamine do not cause cerebral vasoconstriction.[37] In studies of patients with intracranial mass lesions, however, it appeared that although arterial pressure was reduced by 33 percent, cerebral blood volume actually increased secondary to the vasodilatory effect of nitroprusside and was accompanied by an increase in ICP and a decrease in cerebral perfusion pressure.[31] It is therefore suggested that nitroprusside be used cautiously in patients with increased ICP or impaired cerebral autoregulation.[37]

The effects of nitroprusside on CBF and autoregulation are probably influenced by the dose and length of administration as well as the degree of hypotension produced.[37] Loss of autoregulation with prolongation of the vasodilating effect following discontinuance of the drug has been documented, and when arterial pressure was resumed with the use of dopamine, ICP increased for a period of time proportional to the duration of drug administration. It has been hypothesized "that the vasodilatory effect of prolonged nitroprusside administration results in paralysis of vascular smooth muscle, which (after resumption of normal systemic arterial pressure) secondarily results in an increase in cerebral blood volume that is reflected by the increase in intracranial pressure."[36] In addition, the simultaneous administration of a vasopressor (i.e. phenylephrine) may significantly elevate ICP. The nurse should take care to prevent wide swings or fluctuations in blood pressure when administering nitroprusside to neurological patients because of the likelihood of abolishing autoregulation.[39] Monitoring of ICP and calculation of CPP during nitroprusside administration is advisable.

Intravenous nitroglycerine acts primarily by dilating venous capacitance vessels, thereby lowering blood pressure without significantly decreasing cardiac output. Because nitroglycerine acts on the venous capacitance vessels it does not appear to affect autoregulation, and is less likely to increase ICP in patients with intracranial space-occupying lesions.[31] It also has been used to induce controlled hypotension during neurosurgery.[39]

ALTERATIONS AFFECTING THE HEART

Following cerebral insult, reported myocardial alterations include changes in cardiac hemodynamics, dysrhythmias, and histologic and electrocardiographic (ECG) indications of myocardial injury. Cardiac hemodynamic alterations, including chronotropic and inotropic changes, affect arterial blood pressure and consequently CPP and CBF. With severely elevated ICP, the arterial blood pressure increases in an attempt to maintain an adequate CPP, i.e., Cushing's reaction. Likewise, the variability of the heart rate may be affected by neurological injury, and appears to reflect the functional state of the CNS. Normally, the heart rate is not constant, but varies within a certain range in a cyclic fashion during periods of activity and rest. This cycle repeats about every 90–110 minutes, but can vary with the individual. Several factors, including hypoxia, CNS depression, anticholinergic drugs, and age, have been reported to affect cyclic heart rate variability. Similarly, severe CNS injury and increased ICP have been associated with a more constant heart rate. A reduction in the normal cyclic changes in heart rate was verified in a study by Lowensohn et al[40] of ten severely brain-damaged adults. However, they found that return of ICP to normal was not associated with a return of normal heart rate variability until there also was improvement in the clinical neurological status of the patient. The alteration may be due to interruption of the autonomic nervous system influence on the heart caused by injury from elevated ICP, rather than directly to intracranial hypertension. These researches concluded that "the rate of return of variability reflects the subsequent state of neuronal function,"[40] and therefore may be useful in the evaluation of some neurological patients.

The incidence of ECG abnormalities, including dysrhythmias and non-specific ECG changes, has been reported as occurring in up to 80 percent of neurological patients,[41] although the incidence varies greatly in individual studies. ECG abnormalities have been documented in situations where other causes such as preexisting cardiac disease, cardiac drugs, electrolyte disturbances, and blood gas alterations have been ruled out;[21] however, the exact relationship of these changes to the cerebrovascular lesions remains uncertain.

Cardiac Dysrhythmias

Cardiac dysrhythmias have included disturbances of both rhythm and conduction. Atrial and ventricular ectopic impulses, supraventricular tachycardia, atrial fibrillation, sinus tachycardia and bradycardia, as well as atrioventricular (A-V) and bundle branch block have been documented. Life-threatening dysrhythmias, including ventricular tachycardia and fibrillation, have been reported. Subarachnoid hemorrhage has been associated with the highest incidence and most lethal dysrhythmias,[42,43] although a high incidence of ECG changes also has been associated with other acute cerebral lesions and changing ICP.[20,21] Dysrhythmias have occurred following stroke,[30,44] especially resulting from intracerebral hemorrhage.[41,45] Norris et al[30] identified ectopic impulses (supraventricular and ventricular) and atrial fibrillation as the most frequently occurring dysrhythmias in their study of 404 patients admitted to an intensive care stroke unit. Dysrhythmias occurred in 50 percent of the stroke patients with the greatest incidence occurring with lesions of the cerebral hemisphere rather than brainstem.[30] Yamour et al[41] found an increased incidence of dysrhythmias associated with anterior cerebral lesions, although 25 percent of their patients had a sudden development of atrial fibrillation associated with hemorrhage into the brainstem. Clinical experience has shown that stroke victims may die unexpectedly of cardiac arrest or dysrhythmia.[44,46] In patients with cerebral hemorrhage and raised intracranial pressure, Norris et al described common "terminal" rhythms as beginning with a worsening bradycardia and progressing to nodal escape, idioventricular rhythm, and finally cardiac arrest.[30] In addition, there has been a reported case of paroxysmal atrial tachycardia associated with seizure activity, which the authors believe were causally related, in a patient with frontal lobe tumor.[47] ECG changes following head injury have been reported in patients with acute subdural hematoma, and include atrial and ventricular ectopic impulses and rhythms as well as conduction problems.[17] Atrial fibrillation and bundle branch block have occurred and lasted for hours or days following cerebral contusion.[48]

Although dysrhythmias occur more frequently, nonspecific ST and T wave changes have been reported in patients following cerebrovascular hemor-rhage,[41] stroke,[44] subarachnoid hemorrhage,[49] head injury, [48] and elevated ICP.[20] Many of these changes were consistent with cardiac ischemia whether they occurred alone or in association with dysrhythmias.[44] Prominent U waves, ST segment elevation, shortening or prolongation of Q-T intervals, and peaked, notched, or inverted T waves have been observed. "Neurogenic" T waves, seen with various neurological insults, refer to T waves with increased ampli-tude and duration that are also frequently inverted.[50]

Few researchers have ventured hypotheses to explain their clinical find-ings, perhaps because of seemingly inconsistent or contradictory reports on ECG findings. Jachuck et al, however, compared ECG findings with varying levels of ICP and found that: (1) tall T waves may be an early sign of rising ICP but become progressively flatter or invert with ICP above 45 torr; (2) ST segment changes, similar to those seen with myocardial ischemia, occur with changes in ICP rather than structural damage and they return to normal with normalization of the ICP; (3) abnormally shortened QT intervals occur with low levels of elevated ICP while prolongation is associated with ICP over 65 torr.[20]

Documentation of actual myocardial injury associated with neurological disorders is scarce. In an early description of histological cardiac changes following subarachnoid hemorrhage (SAH),[51] the ECGs of 3 subjects prior to death were consistent with subendocardial infarction (i.e., negative T-U fusion waves in multiple leads), and at autopsy, small subendocardial petechial hem-orrhages were found without any significant lesions of the coronary arteries. In 1969, Greenshoot and Reichenbach described microscopic multiple scattered areas of acute myocardial cell injury with disruption of myocardial cell archi-tecture (i.e., myofibrillar degeneration and focal myocytolysis) in 3 patients who died of SAH.[49] Subendocardial interstitial hemorrhage into the left ven-tricle was found in one case. Other studies in humans and animals with sub-arachnoid or intracerebral hemorrhage have reported similar findings.[45,52] The left ventricular subendocardial tissue was most often affected.[20,46] Connor speculated that the infrequent reports of myocardial damage may be because the lesions typically are small and scattered and may be missed unless multiple sections of myocardial tissue are examined at autopsy. He pointed out that histological damage takes time to develop, and therefore myocytolysis is seen only in patients who survive at least 4 to 6 days following the onset of their neurological illness.[46] Development of myocardial damage in patients with intracranial lesions may also be related to autonomic dysfunction. Activation of sympathetic centers, which alters autonomic outflow balance, results in sympathetic discharge capable of producing myocardial necrosis.[49] Myocardial lesions from sympathetic stimulation differ from those in typical myocardial infarction (MI) in that these lesions have been found throughout the heart with apparently normal cells interspersed between abnormal ones; in MI, there is necrosis of all tissue supplied by an affected coronary vessel. In addition, small intracardiac nerves sometimes have been seen immediately adjacent to injured cells with more normal structure at a distance. It has been speculated that myocardial necrosis is secondary to the metabolic effect of norepinephrine released from these nerves into the intracellular space. It was not believed to be due so much to blood-borne catecholamines as these lesions have been found on adrenalectomized animals.[49]

Causes of ECG Changes

Numerous explanations of the causes of the ECG and myocardial changes have been offered. Some authors emphasize that there may be a reason for these cardiac changes that is not directly related to the neurological disorder: (1) underlying hypertension with hypertensive heart disease, (2) previously undiagnosed dysrhythmias, (3) valvular or ischemic heart disease as an etiology for neurological symptoms, (4) generalized atherosclerosis common to both cardiac and cerebral vasculature, (5) other undiagnosed cardiac disease (i.e., cardiomyopathy) and (6) drugs that alter myocardial electrical physiology and hemodynamics. In clinical situations where the above etiologies of ECG changes have been ruled out, neurological changes have been presumed as causative. The effects on the heart of direct stimulation of the sympathetic and parasympathetic systems,[53] stimulation of other areas of the brain,[49] induced increased ICP,[16,21,54] and experimentally produced head trauma and intra-cranial hemorrhage have been studied in laboratory animals.[45,48,55] Both the types of dysrhythmias and histological evidence of cardiac injury in these studies correlate with the observations of patients with intracranial disorders.

As in other cardiovascular changes, the initiation of ECG changes may be mediated by stimulation of the autonomic nervous system directly or by in-creased levels of circulating serum catecholamines,[45,46] although the exact site and pathway of the mechanism is unclear. Weidler suggested that either an increase in autonomic activity or imbalance between the sympathetic and par-asympathetic systems may be the mechanism that produces myocardial damage in subarachnoid hemorrhage.[45] In support of this theory, activation of the sympathetic nervous system peripherally, and intravenous administration of catecholamines in animals produced myocardial damage with subendocardial hemorrhage and focal necrosis. The changes frequently occurred in the inner one-third of the left ventricle and in the papillary muscles. In dog experiments, the injection of isoproterenol in the presence of elevated ICP resulted in cardiac dysrhythmias, including premature atrial and ventricular beats, bursts of ven-tricular tachycardia, and repetitive patterns consisting of a series of rapid beats followed by one or two slow beats.[21] It is postulated that a pathway exists between the cerebral cortex (especially the frontal area) and the hypothalamus to the heart via the sympathetic fibers in the cervical area. This may account for reports of a higher incidence of ECG abnormalities in patients with cerebral hemisphere infarcts[30] and frontal lobe hemorrhages[41] than with brainstem in-juries. Increased vagal tone may be responsible for sinus arrhythmia or bra-dycardia among other dysrhythmias.[21,41] Parasympathetic stimulation via the vagus nerve in dogs has caused ECG changes, signs of cardiac decompensation, and myocardial infarction. Increased parasympathetic activity also may be responsible for similar cardiac changes seen in the critically ill neurological patient. Peptic ulcers, which are commonly seen in these patients, lend clinical evidence for overactivity of the parasympathetic nervous system.[46] Early use of autonomic blockade with such drugs as atropine, reserpine, and propranolol has been advocated for the prevention of the cardiac problems associated with vagal stimulation.[45,53]

The ST-T wave changes suggestive of myocardial ischemia seen in bradycardia may be secondary to altered repolarization caused by autonomic stimulation. It has been shown that alteration of the uniformity in the recovery rate of ventricular myocardial cell excitability (i.e., increase in temporal dispersion in rate of repolarization) may occur with either slow heart rates or sympathetic stimulation.[21] Changes in repolarization are reflected in the S-T segment and T wave on the ECG, and therefore may account for some of the changes seen. Specifically, alteration and delay in ventricular repolarization result in prolongation of the Q-T interval, depression or elevation of the ST segment, tall, peaked, flat, or deeply inverted T waves, and large U waves.[44] In addition, dysrhythmias are more likely to occur with changes in repolarization as disruption in the uniformity of myocardial cell recovery sets the stage for reentrant-type dysrhythmias. Another hypothesis suggests that there may be a "release of neurotransmitter substances into the systemic circulation through the damaged blood-brain barrier."[30] This might account for the fact that increased levels of plasma catecholamines occur with intracranial hemorrhage, and that experimental dysrhythmias produced by cerebral ischemia are prevented by autonomic blockade.[45]

Although alluded to briefly in the literature, no specific studies have been found relating to the stress response following insult to the brain. It is likely that the hypothalamus may be affected in subarachnoid hemorrhage and other neurological disorders and cause a sympathetic outpouring.[53] It has been shown that stress can cause a generalized chain of events, whereby the hypothalamus stimulates the pituitary to secrete ACTH, resulting in the release of catecholamines from the adrenal glands. The heart responds both directly and via the sympathetic nervous system to catecholamines by an increase in its inotropic and chronotropic response, with resultant increase in myocardial oxygen demand. It has been suggested that at the cellular level, depolarization phases of the action potential are altered resulting in electrical instability.[56] These alterations may contribute to the development of dysrhythmias, especially if there is concomitant underlying myocardial disease which disrupts oxygen supply and demand. It has been hypothesized that a severe vasovagal reaction may be the precipitating factor in lethal dysrhythmias with severe psychological stress.[57] Parasympathetic stimulation might also occur with physiological stress in head trauma or other neurological injury, likewise contributing to serious ECG changes.

The incidence and cause of myocardial lesions associated with neurological disorders remains controversial. Subendocardial hemorrhages and myocardial damage are thought to be uncommon, and may correlate with the duration of illness.[49] A transient neurological insult may result in reversible ECG changes, while prolonged periods of neurological injury may cause focal myocardial lesions.[21] If injury to myocardial cells occurs, the development of dysrhythmias may result secondarily from myocardial damage at a cellular or subcellular level.[45]

Clinical Significance of Cardiac Alterations

Impaired circulation adversely influences brain edema or brain damage. A significant reduction in cardiac output can contribute to generalized reduction of CBF and occasionally to focal cerebral ischemia.[30] In addition to deterioration of the patient's neurological status, dysrhythmias have been associated with new cerebral embolization in up to 17 percent of stroke patients.[30] In a study of patients with acute subdural hematoma, it was found that dysrhythmias such as premature ventricular beats were often precursors of more serious ventricular dysrhythmias, such as ventricular tachycardia and ventricular fibrillation (12 of 17 patients).[17] In neurosurgical units, patients without preexisting heart lesions or blood loss have died of dysrhythmias, cardiac arrest, or severe hypotension.[46]

Lavy et al demonstrated a poor prognosis in stroke patients with coexisting cardiac abnormalities.[44] In addition, it has been found that patients with abnormal ECGs have a higher mortality rate than other patients. In patients with acute subdural hematoma, it has been speculated that either ECG changes are a poor prognostic sign or the severely injured patient is more likely to develop an ECG abnormality.[17] This would certainly emphasize the importance of close attention to cardiac monitoring of the head-injured patient, with reporting and follow-up care of dysrhythmias. Hearts for transplantation are generally recovered from patients dying of cerebrovascular disease or head injury. In light of the possibility that myocardial damage may result from intracranial pathology, it has been suggested that some of these patients may no longer be considered suitable donors.[53]

CONCLUSION

Maintenance of adequate cerebral circulation is vital to preservation of neurological function. Direct injury to the brain may alter cerebral blood flow either focally or globally thereby complicating the clinical course of a patient with an already compromised neurological status. Insufficient CBF will result in cerebral ischemia, while an increase in CBF may contribute to cerebral edema. In order to understand how and why these changes occur, it is essential to be aware of autoregulation and the effect of the autonomic nervous system on regulation of CBF, and the factors that interfere with the normal delicate balance in cerebral circulation. Loss of normal regulatory mechanisms makes the cerebral vasculature susceptible to outside influences and can result in unusual shifts of blood within the brain. Although usually complicating the initial injury, occasionally these changes have been utilized in medical treatment in an attempt to improve the circulatory status of the brain. Injury to the brain also has been associated with alterations in cardiac hemodynamics and the development of dysrhythmias. Electrocardiographic and histologic evidence of myocardial injury has been reported. Realizing that some of these changes may have clinical significance emphasizes the importance of frequent monitoring of cardiovascular status in the early management of patients with intracranial injury.[48,53] Correlation of cardiovascular changes with other clinical changes and monitored neurological parameters may ultimately aid the assessment and care of these patients.

REFERENCES

1. Bucy C: Neurosurgical nursing. Editorial, Surg Neurol 6:61, 1976.
2. McHenry L, Toole J, Miller H: Long-term EKG monitoring in patients with cerebrovascular insufficiency. Stroke 7:264–269, 1976.
3. Goldberg AD, Raftery EB, Cashman PM: Ambulatory electrocardiographic records in patients with transient cerebral attacks or palpitation. Br Med J 6 Dec: 569–571, 1975.
4. Plum F, Posner JB: The diagnosis of stupor and coma. Contemporary Neurology Series. 3rd edition, FA Davis Co., Philadelphia, 1980.
5. Scheinberg P: Cerebral blood flow. In Tower DB, Chase TN, Eds: The Nervous System Vol 2: Clinical Neurosciences, Raven Press, New York, 1975.
6. Overgaard J, Tweed WA: Studies of regional cerebral blood flow. In Trubuhovich RV, Ed: International Anesthesiology Clinics: Management of Acute Intracranial Disasters Vol. 17, pp. 413–424. Little, Brown and Company, Boston, 1979.
7. MacKenzie ET, Farrar JK, Fitch W, Graham D, Gregory PC, Harper AM: Effects of hemorrhagic hypotension on the cerebral circulation. Stroke 10:711–718, 1979.
8. Shapiro HM: Intracranial hypertension: Therapeutic and anesthetic considerations. Anesthesiology 43:433–469, 1975.
9. Purves MJ: Control of cerebral blood vessels: Present state of the art. Annals of Neurology 3:337–383, 1978.
10. Guyton AC: Textbook of Medical Physiology. WB Saunders, Philadelphia, 1976.
11. McGillicuddy JE, Kindt GW, Raisis JE, Miller CA: The relation of cerebral ischemia, hypoxia, and hypercarbia to the Cushing response. J Neurosurg 48:730–740. 1978.
12. Quint S, Schremin O, Sonnenschein R, Rubinstein E: Enhancement of cerebrovascular effect of CO_2 by hypoxia. Stroke 11:286, 1980.
13. Borgstrom L, Johnson H, Siesjö B: The relationship between arterial PO_2 and cerebral blood flow in hypoxic hypoxia. Acta Physiol Scand 93:423–432, 1975.
14. Siesjö BK, Nordstrom CH, Rehncrona S: Metabolic aspects of cerebral hypoxia-ischemia. Adv in Exp Med & Bio 78:261–269, 1977.
15. Miller JD, Sullivan HG: Severe intracranial hypertension. In Trubuhovich, RV, Ed: International Anesthesiology Clinics: Management of Acute Intracranial Disasters Vol 17. pp. 19–75, Little Brown and Co, Boston, Summer-Fall, 1979.
16. Miner ME, Gonzalez NC, Overman J: Cardiovascular response to independent cephalic and spinal cord pressure elevations. Surgical Forum 23:407–409, 1972.
17. VanderArk GD: Cardiovascular changes with acute subdural hematoma. Surg Neurol 3:305–308, 1975.

18. Marshall LF, Smith RW, Shapiro HM: The influence of diurnal rhythms in patients with intracranial hypertension: Implications for management. Neurosurgery 2:100–102, 1978.
19. Schneider RC: Craniocerebral trauma. In Kahn EA, Crosby EC, Schneider RC, Taren, JA, Eds: Correlative Neurosurgery. Charles C Thomas, Springfield, 1969.
20. Jachuck SJ, Ramani PS, Clark F, Kalbag: Electrocardiographic abnormalities associated with raised intracranial pressure. Br Med J 1:242–244, 1975.
21. Smith M, Ray C: Cardiac arrhythmias, increased intracranial pressure, and the autonomic nervous system. Chest 61:125–133, 1972.
22. Langfitt TW: Increased intracranial pressure. Clinical Neurosurgery 16:436–471, 1969.
23. Enevoldsen EM, Jensen FT: Autoregulation and CO_2 responses of cerebral blood flow in patients with acute severe head injury. J. Neurosurg 48:689–703, 1978.
24. Ginsburg D, Reivich M: Cerebrovascular pathophysiology. In Chase TN, Tower DB, Eds: The Nervous System Vol. 2: Clinical Neurosciences. Raven Press, New York, 1975.
25. Ignelzi R: Cerebral edema: Present perspectives. Neurosurgery 4:338–342, 1979.
26. Hoff JT: Resuscitation in focal brain ischemia. Crit Care Med 6:245–252, 1978.
27. Safar P: Introduction: On the evolution of brain resuscitation. Crit Care Med 6:199–202, 1978.
28. Safar P, Bleyaert A, Nemoto EM, Moossy J, Snyder J: Resuscitation after global brain ischemia-anoxia. Crit Care Med 6:215–227, 1978.
29. Nemoto EM: Pathogenesis of cerebral ischemia-anoxia. Crit Care Med 6:203–214, 1978.
30. Norris JW, Froggatt GM, Hachinski VC: Cardiac arrhythmias in acute stroke. Stroke 9:392–396, 1978.
31. Cottrell JE, Patel K, Turndorf H, Ransohoff J: Intracranial pressure changes induced by sodium nitroprusside in patients with intracranial mass lesions. J Neurosurg 48:329–331, 1978.
32. Janzer RC, Friede RL: Perisulcal infarcts: Lesions caused by hypotension during increased intracranial pressure. Annals of Neurology 6:399–404, 1979.
33. Shapiro HM: Intracranial hypertension: Therapeutic and anesthetic considerations. Anesthesiology 43:433–469, 1975.
34. Schmidek H: Subarachnoid hemorrhage. In Oaks W, Bharadwaja K, Major DA, Eds: Critical Care: The Fortieth Hahnemann Symposium. Grune and Stratton, New York, 1978.
35. Allen GS, Gross CJ: Cerebral arterial spasm: Part 7, Surg Neurol 6:63–80, 1976.
36. Weiss MH, Spence J, Apuzzo M, Heiden JS, McComb G, Kurze T: Influence of nitroprusside on cerebral pressure autoregulation. Neurosurgery 4:56–59, 1979.
37. Candia GJ, Heros R, Lavyne M, Zervas N, Nelson C: Effect of intravenous sodium nitroprusside on cerebral blood flow and intracranial pressure. Neurosurgery 3:50–52, 1978.
38. Griffiths DPG, Gummins BH, Greenbaum R, Griffiths HB, Staddon GE, Wilkins DG, Zorab JSM: Cerebral blood flow and metabolism during hypotension induced with sodium nitroprusside. Br J Anaesth 46:671–679, 1974.
39. Chestnut JS, Albin MS, Gonzalez-Abola E, Maroon JC: Clinical evaluation of intravenous nitroglycerin for neurosurgery. J Neurosurg 48:704–711, 1978.
40. Lowensohn RI, Weiss M, Hon H: Heart-rate variability in brain-damaged adults. The Lancet 1:626–628, 1977.

41. Yamour BJ, Sridharan MR, Rice JF, Flowers NC: Electrocardiographic changes in cerebrovascular hemorrhage. Am Heart J 99:294–300, 1980.
42. Parizel G: Life-threatening arrhythmias in subarachnoid hemorrhage. Angiology 24:17–21, 1973.
43. Estanol BV, Marin OS: Cardiac arrhythmias and sudden death in subarachnoid hemorrhage. Stroke 6:382–386, 1975.
44. Lavy S, Yaar I, Melamed E: The effect of acute stroke on cardiac functions as observed in an intensive stroke care unit. Stroke 5:775–780, 1974.
45. Weidler DJ: Myocardial damage and cardiac arrhymias after intracranial hemorrhage: A critical review. Stroke 5:759–764, 1974.
46. Connor R: Myocardial damage secondary to brain lesions. Am Heart J 78:145–148, 1969.
47. Rush J, Everett B, Adams A, Kusske J: Paroxysmal atrial tachycardia and frontal lobe tumor. Arch Neurol 34:578–580, 1977.
48. McLaurin RL, King LR: Recognition and treatment of metabolic disorders after head injuries. Clinical Neurosurgery 19:281–300, 1971.
49. Greenhoot JH, Reichenbach DD: Cardiac injury and subarachnoid hemorrhage. J Neurosurg 30:521–531, 1969.
50. Burch GE, Meyers R, Abildskov JA: A new electrocardiographic pattern observed in cerebrovascular accidents. Circulation 9:719–723, 1954.
51. Koskelo P, Punsar S, Sipila W: Subendocardial hemorrhage and ECG changes in intracranial bleeding. Br Med J 1:1479–1480, 1964.
52. Connor R: Heart damage associated with intracranial lesions. Br Med J 3:29, 1968.
53. Weintraub B, McHenry L: Cardiac abnormalities in subarachnoid hemorrhage: A resume. Stroke 5:384–392, 1974.
54. VanderArk GD, Norton LW, Pomerantz M: Cardiovascular effects of increased intracranial pressure. Surgical Forum 23:409–411, 1972.
55. Hawkins WE, Clower BR: Myocardial damage after head trauma and simulated intracranial hemorrhage in mice: The role of the autonomic nervous system. CV Research 5:524–529, 1971.
56. Wit A, Hoffman B, Rosen M: Electrophysiology and pharmacology of cardiac arrhythmias. Am Heart J 90:521–533, 1975.
57. Engel G: Psychological stress, vasodepressor syndrome and sudden death. Annals of Int Med 89:403–412, 1978.

4 | Respiratory Complications of Intracranial Disorders

Sarah J. Sanford

One of the many critical functions of the central nervous system is to assure that ventilation is appropriate to overall physiologic need. Because the nature of this task is complex, disruption of the interactions involved in neurogenic control of respiration is likely to occur in the presence of intracranial pathology. Not surprisingly, such pathology is frequently associated with respiratory dysfunction. Alterations in the amount of circulating oxygen and carbon dioxide can result from dysfunction, and, if severe, can increase damage to an already compromised central nervous system. As a framework for the discussion of respiratory dysfunction in intracranial disorders, a review of nervous system interactions involved in initiation and control of ventilation is presented.

NEUROGENIC COORDINATION OF BREATHING

Breathing requires rhythmic and integrated contraction and relaxation of inspiratory and expiratory respiratory muscles. While the inspiratory phase is associated with contraction of inspiratory muscles, expiration most frequently reflects passive elastic recoil of the chest wall and lungs. When active expiration is necessary, coordinated contraction of expiratory muscles also must occur. Smooth transition between the two phases of respiration is coordinated in

73

respiratory centers, specialized areas of the brainstem. While there is general agreement as to the identity and location of the respiratory centers, their precise functions are still being defined.

Brainstem Respiratory Centers

The most caudal of the three respiratory centers is the *medullary respiratory center*. Located in the reticular formation of the medulla oblongata, this center is functionally composed of inspiratory and expiratory neurons.[1,2] Impulses initiated by the two types of neurons are transmitted down the spinal cord to their respective effector muscles.[1,2] Impulse generation from the medullary respiratory center is inherently rhythmic and while reciprocal inhibition by the two types of neurons does occur, functionally the expiratory neurons operate primarily in situations requiring active expiration.[1] Most commonly, the inspiratory neurons are dominant and their discharge in a characteristically cyclic pattern establishes rhythmicity.[1]

The two other brainstem respiratory centers are located in the pons. Both pontine centers affect the action of the medullary center although in relatively opposite ways. The *apneustic* center in the pontine reticular formation is linked by an extensive network of interneurons to the inspiratory neurons of the medulla.[2] Generally, it is inspirostimulatory, that is, activation of the apneustic center initiates an inspiratory effort.[1] The vagus nerve directly innervates the apneustic center and is generally inhibitory. Vagal stimulation, therefore, is associated with slowed frequency of inspiratory effort, giving the appearance of enhanced or prolonged expiration; presumably the vagal effect is a function of apneustic center inhibition.[1] The vagus is functionally a component of several proprioceptive reflex pathways that affect ventilation and are discussed in a later section.

The *pneumotaxic center* is the second pontine respiratory center. Extensive interneuronal connections link it to the apneustic center and probably to the medullary center as well.[1,2] The pneumotaxic center is functionally thought to terminate inspiratory activity and thus is generally inhibitory to the medullary inspiratory center.[1] Sources of input to the pneumotaxic center have not been well defined, although it is thought that neuronal discharge by the medullary inspiratory center initiates pneumotaxic activity and in that way serves to assure smooth transition between the inspiratory and expiratory phases of the respiratory cycle.

Evidence from animal studies indicates that the respiratory cycle reflects a balance between tonic inhibitory influence upon brainstem centers by the cerebral cortex and tonic facilatory influences from the hypothalamus and other diencephalic structures.[3–5] Evidence is based on experimental studies in which animals have been subjected to cortical or brainstem damage and the observation that hyperventilatory syndromes follow diffuse cortical damage while hypoventilatory syndromes follow severe brainstem damage.[3–5] However, the mechanisms of cortical inhibition and brainstem facilitation are not clear and the reader is referred to the section on abnormal breathing patterns for further discussion.

The respiratory pattern produced by the brainstem respiratory centers is relatively automatic in that voluntary desire to breath is not necessary for its occurrence. However, voluntary alteration of the respiratory pattern is possible and cerebral cortical influence can, to a limited extent, dominate the activity of the brainstem respiratory centers. Such is the case in voluntary breathholding and speaking.

Modification of breathing also occurs in conjunction with emotional reactions and reflex activities such as swallowing and gagging.[1] Intense emotions such as fear and anger are associated with an overall increase in respiratory rate as well as use of ancillary muscles normally not employed in the respiratory cycle.[1] The mechanism involved in these cases is not clear but is thought to involve functional connection between the respiratory centers, cranial nerves, and centers of autonomic activity.

Alteration of the inherent rhythmicity of the medullary respiratory center occurs when nonrespiratory sensory neurons stimulate discharge of respiratory neurons.[1,2] These nonrespiratory neurons produce inspiratory neuronal discharge in response to relatively nonspecific stimuli such as pain, heat, and cold. The traditional spanking of newborns and the subsequent inspiratory gasp is an example of this mechanism.

Humoral/Chemical Feedback

Regulation of pulmonary ventilation also occurs as a result of specific humoral and chemical stimuli, as well as proprioceptive reflexes.[1,2]

Metabolic processes continually alter carbon dioxide (CO_2) production, oxygen (O_2) consumption and the pH of body fluids. Such continuous chemical alterations require that pulmonary ventilation be dynamically adjusted to ensure homeostatic balance.

Carbon dioxide is the most potent naturally occurring stimulus to pulmonary ventilation.[1] Changes in circulating CO_2 tension (PCO_2) as small as 2 to 3 torr produce a measurable increase in ventilation.[2] Chemoreceptors on the ventrolateral surface of the medulla, sensitive to both CO_2 and hydrogen ion (H^+), are believed to be involved in the ventilatory response to hypercapnia.[1] Diffusion of CO_2 across the blood-brain barrier is relatively unimpeded and its entrance into the cerebrospinal fluid (CSF) results in stimulation of the central chemoreceptors.[1] Ideally, the subsequent increase in ventilation lowers blood PCO_2 and, through equilibration, the CSF CO_2 tension as well.

Carbon dioxide in the CSF reacts with water (H_2O) to form carbonic acid which dissociates to bicarbonate ion (HCO_3^-) and hydrogen ion (H^+). However, because CSF content of the catalytic enzyme carbonic anhydrase is relatively low, formation of HCO_3^- and H^+ proceeds relatively slowly. Therefore there is a delay before the CO_2 which enters the CSF results in production of significant quantities of H^+.[1,2] Because of this time lag it is most likely that

CSF CO_2 tension and not H^+ content is the primary stimulating factor for the central chemoreceptors in hypercapnia.

Buffering capacity of the CSF is less than that of blood, primarily because of a lesser content of protein.[1] The blood-brain barrier is normally relatively impermeable to H^+ and HCO_3^-, thus changes in blood pH are not immediately reflected in the CSF pH. However, in the presence of local H^+ production, as occurs in cerebral ischemia or excessive cerebral metabolic activity, permeability to H^+ ions is increased, facilitating diffusion into the CSF.[1] The result can be a substantial decrease in the pH of the CSF. While the mechanism behind altered H^+ permeability is not clear, in situations of local H^+ production, it may be the H^+ that produces stimulation of the medullary chemoreceptors and the subsequent increase in pulmonary ventilation.[1]

A secondary set of chemoreceptors sensitive to CO_2 are located in the angle of the bifurcation of the common carotid arteries and in the aortic arch.[1,2] These peripheral chemoreceptors increase their stimulatory impulses to the medullary respiratory center whenever blood that perfuses them has a PCO_2 greater than 40 torr. In fact, increased ventilation in hypercapneic states is probably initiated by the peripheral chemoreceptors.[1] Despite the fact that central chemoreceptors are more sensitive to CO_2 than their peripheral counterparts, central chemoreceptor activation is slower because diffusion across the blood-brain barrier must first occur. However, once activated, central chemoreceptors are thought to be responsible for the sustained increase in ventilation.

Hypoxemia stimulates peripheral chemoreceptors to increase pulmonary ventilation, but the arterial oxygen tension must fall to about 50 torr before ventilation increases.[1,2] Under normal conditions, the degree of ventilation regulation provided by this mechanism is probably secondary to that resulting from blood pH changes. This is evidenced by the fact that hypoxemia-induced hyperventilation reduces the PCO_2, increases the blood pH, and consequently inhibits further ventilatory response to hypoxemia.[1,2] However, both the sensitivity threshold of the peripheral chemoreceptors and the ventilatory response produced in hypoxemia is increased by concomitant hypercapnia.[2] Because of this interaction, the hypoxic mechanism for physiologic regulation of ventilation is important; indeed, in the presence of chronic pulmonary insufficiency it is probably the primary regulatory mechanism.[1]

While hypercapnia increases ventilation via stimulation of both peripheral and central chemoreceptors, hypoxemia stimulates only the former.[2] If the peripheral chemoreceptors are denervated, as can occur in bilateral carotid endarterectomy, the hypoxic drive can be lost. In addition, because hypoxia has a direct depressant effect on the brainstem respiratory center, extreme care is needed when administering pharmacologic agents that have respiratory depressant effects to these patients.[2]

Metabolic acidosis and increased H^+ concentration profoundly stimulate pulmonary ventilation, but as previously discussed, probably not as a function of alteration of the CSF pH.[1,2] Peripheral chemoreceptors are sensitive to increased H^+ but the hyperventilatory response to acidosis occurs even when these receptors have been denervated.[1,2] While not clearly defined, the ventilatory response to acidosis is thought to involve some additional mechanism, possibly a direct effect on the H^+ ions on the medullary center.[1]

Proprioceptive Reflexes

Receptors for several proprioceptive reflexes are located in the lungs and chest wall. The sensory pathways from most of these receptors travel to the brainstem via the vagus nerve to influence the respiratory pattern. There are many such reflexes but only three will be discussed here.

The inspiroinhibitory reflex, also known as the Hering-Breuer reflex, affects the depth of inspiration.[2] Stretch receptors known as Hering-Breuer receptors are located throughout the lung, bronchi, and bronchioles and are stimulated by lung inflation and airway distention, which may occur when exhalation is impeded. Under normal conditions, the threshold for receptor activation seems to be relatively high, requiring a tidal volume of at least a full liter.[2] However, in situations of decreased lung compliance or increased airway resistance, the sensitivity of the Hering-Breuer receptors is increased.[1] Receptor stimulation causes inhibition of inspiration and prolongation of expiration.[2] Presumably, activation of this reflex inhibits the apneustic center (normally inspirostimulatory) which is known to be inhibited by the vagus, but a direct medullary center affect has not been disproved.

Juxtacapillary receptors, or J receptors, are located near the pulmonary capillaries and are stimulated by increased interstitial fluid volume or pulmonary congestion.[2,3] Activation of these receptors is thought to initiate transmission of impulses along sensory vagal fibers.[3] Presumably, the frequency of impulses defines the response, which varies from apnea to tachypnea. While precise frequency-response relationships have not been defined, it appears that as pulmonary congestion or interstitial fluid volume increases so does the respiratory rate, until at some highly individual point the increased volume/congestion depresses the drive to the point of apnea.[3]

The third reflex involves epithelial irritant receptors which are stimulated by bronchial or bronchiolar congestion or mechanical irritation producing tachypnea and bronchoconstriction.[2,3]

Decreased pulmonary compliance, bronchial, interstitial, or pulmonary congestion can occur as a function of intracranial pathology. Therefore, although the role(s) of these reflex mechanisms is not entirely clear, they probably contribute, at least in part, to the production of abnormalities in breathing patterns commonly seen in central nervous system insult.

ABNORMAL RESPIRATORY PATTERNS IN CENTRAL NERVOUS SYSTEM DISORDERS

A variety of abnormal breathing patterns result from central nervous system malfunctions that interfere with either the neurogenesis of normal breathing or the integration of the various factors involved in the respiratory drive. While normal respiratory patterns do occur in the presence of intracranial pathology, such pathology is usually limited to small unilateral lesions.[2]

Cheyne-Stokes Breathing

Periodic breathing in which hyperpnea regularly alternates with apnea is known as Cheyne-Stokes breathing. In this pattern of respiration, the depth of inspiration increases from breath to breath in a smooth crescendo, then decreases in depth in an equally smooth decrescendo until an apneic phase occurs.[1,6] The hyperpneic phase is usually longer than the apneic phase. It is postulated that an abnormally increased ventilatory response to carbon dioxide, as part of an overall decreased cortical modulation of all chemoreflexes, is involved in the mechanism behind Cheyne-Stokes respirations.[6-8]

Clinically, Cheyne-Stokes respirations are associated with bilateral cerebral hemispheric lesions or lesions of the basal ganglia caused by extensive cerebral vascular disease and/or hypertensive encephalopathies.[3,6] This pattern also may accompany metabolic encephalopathies, such as uremia.[6] Emergence of the Cheyne-Stokes pattern in the presence of traumatic supratentorial lesions is ominous as it is usually indicative of impending tentorial herniation. Cheyne-Stokes respirations are usually accompanied by unconsciousness and decorticate responses to painful stimuli.[6,9]

Central Neurogenic Hyperventilation

Lesions of the midbrain and pons, as the result of cerebral infarcts or trauma, have been implicated in producing a respiratory pattern characterized by sustained, regular, rapid, and fairly deep hyperpnea. Occurrence of this respiratory pattern, known as central neurogenic hyperventilation, markedly decreases the arterial CO_2 tension leading to respiratory alkalosis. Because alkalosis, through a direct vasoconstrictive effect, is known to reduce cerebral blood flow and consequently intracranial pressure, such hyperventilation is viewed by some as compensatory response to intracranial hypertension.[3]

In the presence of increased intracranial pressure, decreased cerebral perfusion may lead to development of CSF lactic acidosis. Because central chemoreceptors are highly sensitive to H^+ in the CSF, such acidosis could theoretically initiate central neurogenic hyperventilation. The additive effect of respiratory alkalosis and subsequent cerebral vasoconstriction would then serve to perpetuate cerebral ischemia, CSF lactic acidosis, and stimulation of the central chemoreceptors. Indeed, studies on head-injured and stroke patients have demonstrated the existence of CSF lactic acidosis in those patients with this type of hyperventilation.[10]

While the central chemoreceptor role in initiating central neurogenic hyperventilation is plausible, many believe the CSF lactic acidosis is a secondary rather than primary event.[3,10] There is also some question as to the role that CSF H^+ content actually plays in the regulation of pulmonary ventilation in man, especially in situations where arterial and thus CSF CO_2 tension is decreased.[11] A humoral mechanism, therefore, has been postulated in central neurogenic hyperventilation. Specifically, increase in circulating catecholamines and fatty acids, both known to induce hyperventilation, have been implicated.[12-14] In sudden central nervous system disruptions, the physiologic stress response is evoked, leading to sympathetic nervous system stimulation and elevations in the circulating levels of both these substances.[2,10,16] Additionally, it is not unlikely that the production and release of catecholamines and neurotransmitters by the central nervous system is altered by intracranial insult.[2,16]

Excessive sympathetic stimulation also produces primary pulmonary changes that include subclinical pulmonary congestion, increased interstitial fluid volume, and decreased pulmonary compliance.[19,20] These changes will be discussed in detail in a later section but it is significant that all three are capable of initiating tachypnea via proprioceptive reflex pathways.

Finally, impaired cortical inhibition of brainstem centers has been causally implicated in central neurogenic hyperventilation. Historically, this respiratory pattern has been linked with traumatic "brainstem contusion," leading to the assumption that isolated brainstem injury is responsible. However, recent clinical investigation indicates that such classification of injury is probably incorrect because in the presence of such an injury, concomitant diffuse supratentorial microhemorrhage is extremely likely.[3,17-20] Computerized axial tomography studies, as well as pathological studies of individuals so injured, have failed to demonstrate isolated brainstem changes without coexisting generalized damage throughout the hemispheres.[18-20] When this respiratory pattern occurs in traumatic injury, it is usually associated with decerebrate rigidity, thus giving further credence to the existence of "higher" abnormalities.[17-20] The emergence of central neurogenic hyperventilation is probably a function of interaction between several mechanisms which at present have not been totally defined.

Apneustic Breathing

Sustained, cramplike, inspiratory efforts only irregularly interrupted by brief expirations are characteristic of apneustic breathing. It is a rare occurrence and usually accompanies basilar artery occlusion and mid to caudal pontine infarction; it may also accompany severe meningitis, hypoxemia, and hypoglycemia.[2,6] This respiratory pattern represents the uninhibited effect of the apneustic center upon medullary inspiratory neurons.[1] Normally, the higher pneumotaxic center modifies apneustic activity and facilitates smooth inspiratory to expiratory transition.

Ataxic Breathing

Ataxic respirations are completely irregular, consisting of both deep and shallow inspiratory efforts. Their emergence is usually evidence of irreversible and terminal central nervous system dysfunction and are due to primary disruption of the inspiratory and expiratory components of the medullary respiratory center.[2,6] Frequently, an ataxic breathing pattern progresses to complete apnea. Medullary compression in herniation syndromes as well as expanding posterior fossa lesions are typically the pathologies producing ataxic breathing.[6,9]

Respiratory Changes Associated with Herniation Syndromes

In central nervous system pathology involving progressive increases in intracranial pressure leading to cerebral herniation, the respiratory pattern generally reflects compression of intracranial structures in a fairly predictable way. Excessive yawning and sighing in the presence of central herniation syndrome is thought to reflect early hypothalamic and thalamic pressure, but may also be a function of an overall increase in drowsiness due to the increasing intracranial pressure.[6] The Cheyne-Stokes respiratory pattern in progressively increasing intracranial pressure is generally indicative of pronounced diencephalic pressure with central herniation and is most commonly accompanied by decorticate responses to pain, a decreased level of consciousness, and small but reactive pupils.[6,9] As increased intracranial pressure continues, the appearance of central neurogenic hyperventilation is usually reflective of herniation of the uncus of the temporal lobe over the edge of the tentorium, causing compression of the midbrain and upper pons. This is usually associated with an ipsilateral dilated and fixed pupil.[6,9] With further compression of the brainstem in both herniation syndromes, decerebrate responses to pain, nonreactive, midposition pupils, and sluggish or absent oculocephalic reflexes accompany central neurogenic hyperventilation.[6,9] Medullary compression is reflected by development of flaccid paralysis and is usually accompanied by ataxic respirations; these findings usually signal a progression of pathology that is both irreversible and terminal.[6]

PULMONARY PATHOPHYSIOLOGY IN INTRACRANIAL DISORDERS

Pulmonary insufficiency associated with insult confined to the central nervous system is not a rare event.[15,21] Although the precise mechanisms of pulmonary insufficiency caused by intracranial disorders have not been clearly defined, there is clearly a relationship.[16,23]

Development of extreme ventilation/perfusion mismatch (V/Q mismatch) or "*shunt*" associated with hypoxemia is a common form of pulmonary dysfunction in patients with severe head injuries.[16,21–26] A "mismatch" involving perfusion of poorly ventilated or nonventilated alveoli, or ventilation of alveoli having compromised perfusion, or a combination of the two, creates V/Q inequality.[16,21,22] V/Q mismatch has been noted in these patients even when other causes such as pneumonia, pneumonitis, pneumothorax, cardiac insufficiency, and fluid overload, have been excluded.[16]

A common denominator of ventilation/perfusion mismatch in head-injured patients is increased intracranial pressure.[22] In severe head injury, increased intracranial pressure is accompanied by stimulation of the sympathetic nervous system.[2,24] Data from animal experiments suggest that intense sympathetic discharge decreases pulmonary compliance by altering surfactants.[27,28] Such changes are capable of initiating microatelectasis, although studies measuring functional residual capacity in individuals with V/Q mismatch have not indicated that atelectasis is present to a significant degree.[16] In addition, institution of positive pressure ventilation with correction of hypoxemia has not corrected the mismatch.[16,22,23,25,26] While subclinical atelectasis could exist, it apparently is not the primary mechanism in development of V/Q mismatch and hypoxemia in intracranial disorders.

Intense sympathetic discharge has additional effects which may be involved in the development of ventilation/perfusion disorders. Initially, adrenergic stimulation with subsequent peripheral vasoconstriction and increased peripheral vascular resistance forces blood into the relatively low resistance pulmonary circuit.[16,29,30] This increase in volume results in increased pulmonary capillary pressure and pulmonary hypertension.[23,29,30] Additionally, intense sympathetic discharge causes pulmonary vasoconstriction, which eventually affects pulmonary venules as well as pulmonary arterioles.[23] The combination of increased volume in the pulmonary circuit and venular constriction is thought to produce capillary trapping of blood and subsequent distention of the microvasculature.[23] Such distention is damaging to the vessels, and coupled with the increased hydrostatic pressure from increased pulmonary blood volume, causes fluid extravasation into the interstitium and alveoli.[23,29,30] If the sympathetic discharge is prolonged, *neurogenic pulmonary edema* results and proceeds to progressive congestive atelectasis, respiratory failure, and a syndrome difficult to differentiate from adult respiratory distress syndrome.

Animal studies have suggested that pharmacologic agents may have value in the prevention of neurogenic respiratory problems. Reports of findings in experimental settings indicate that pulmonary compromise following inflicted cerebral insult has been minimized with sympathetic alpha blockade. Phenoxybenzamine, administered prior to cerebral insult, has been reported to reduce the sympathetically-mediated increase in peripheral and pulmonary vascular resistance believed to be responsible for development of neurogenic pulmonary edema.[29,30] Phenytoin (Dilantin) may also alter the sympathetic discharge in acute head injuries, although the mechanism involved is obscure.[23] Central nervous system depressants, including phenobarbital, ether, and chloral hydrate, have also been documented as decreasing neurogenic pulmonary edema when administered prior to inflicting cerebral insult.[29] While these findings offer encouragement, it is not known what effect these agents would have on humans who have already experienced cerebral insult at the time of administration.

Clinically, neurogenic pulmonary edema is a relatively rare occurrence in individuals hospitalized for severe head injuries.[16,29,30] Studies in which pulmonary vascular pressures have been monitored in head-injured patients indicate that pulmonary hypertension does not often accompany pulmonary V/Q mismatch and hypoxemia.[22,25,26] It is important to note, however, that individuals with severe head injuries are routinely and vigorously treated with fluid restriction and diuretics in an effort to decrease intracranial pressure. Successful lowering of intracranial pressure, known to decrease the sympathetic discharge, and concomitant fluid restriction, probably limit the development of pulmonary vascular distention and elevation of pulmonary vascular pressures.[23] However, limiting the period of pulmonary distention does not preclude the possibility that the initial sympathetic discharge and consequent pulmonary changes could produce pulmonary capillary damage that, although not manifested clinically as adult respiratory distress syndrome, does impair pulmonary capillary autoregulatory mechanisms.[22,23] For example, impairment of the hypoxic pulmonary capillary vasoconstrictive response coupled with microatelectasis could explain the development of V/Q mismatch and hypoxemia, even in the absence of clinical pulmonary edema or adult respiratory distress syndrome.

It should be assumed that all head-injured patients are hypoxemic until proven otherwise.[24,25] Severe hypoxemia (oxygen tension less than 50 torr) produces cerebral vasodilatation, increased intracranial pressure, and cerebral hypoxia.[25,31] However, even if hypoxemia is not severe enough to result in cerebral vasodilatation, the potential for aggravation of existing cerebral hypoxia remains.[24,25,31] Additionally, cerebral hypoxia is capable of initiating autonomically mediated pulmonary venular spasm and therefore V/Q mismatch.[16,23] If not corrected, hypoxemia potentiates cerebral hypoxia and may initiate a vicious circle of progressive pulmonary and neurologic deterioration. Research has documented that V/Q mismatch and hypoxemia not only occur immediately after intracranial insult but on a delayed basis as well; in fact, hypoxemia has been found to increase in severity 24 hours after insult, and for periods lasting 3 to 5 days.[16,24-26]

The need for initial and serial arterial blood gas analysis is critical for identifying and correcting hypoxemia. Tracheal intubation may be required to ensure that the airway is unobstructed. Supplemental oxygen, possibly with mechanical ventilatory assistance, should be standard in the initial resuscitation of head-injured patients.

Iatrogenic hyperventilation with maintenance of an arterial CO_2 tension of 25–30 torr is frequently initiated in patients with intracranial insult.[15] Hyperventilation with large tidal volumes may facilitate alveolar expansion, thereby decreasing any contributory role of atelectasis in ventilation-perfusion defects. Decreased arterial CO_2 levels causes vasoconstriction, decreases cerebral blood flow, and consequently intracranial pressure.[3] However, arterial CO_2 tensions less than 25 torr introduce the risk of decreasing cerebral blood flow to the point of producing cerebral ischemia and CSF lactic acidosis.[3,10] Excessive hyperventilation that is accompanied by cerebral hypoxia directly impairs cellular mechanisms that control intracellular water volume, and may therefore lead to cerebral edema and increased intracranial pressure.[9,16] Because of the danger of aggravation of intracranial hypertension, many support the use of intracranial pressure monitoring for comatose patients in whom iatrogenic hyperventilation is employed.[16,26,30] Through monitoring of intracranial pressure the arterial CO_2 tension associated with the lowest mean intracranial pressure can be determined.

If neurogenic pulmonary edema and/or adult respiratory distress syndrome develop, additional measures for maximizing alveolar-capillary gas exchange are required. Continuous positive pressure ventilation, supplemental oxygen, aggressive secretion management, serial blood gas and chest x-ray analysis, fluid restriction, and administration of hyperosmolar agents and diuretics are standard components in the treatment of such syndromes.[23] Positive end-expiratory pressure (PEEP) may also be used to maintain adequate arterial oxygen tensions; however, its use is not without controversy. No doubt exists as to the efficacy of PEEP in improving arterial oxygenation while simultaneously limiting the fraction of inspired oxygen; however, the neurologic effects are thought by some to outweigh the benefits.

PEEP increases intrathoracic pressure, which may increase central venous pressure, decrease venous return, and therefore decrease cardiac output.[33,35,37] These hemodynamic changes can result in decreased systemic blood pressure.[35] In the presence of intracranial hypertension, cerebral perfusion pressure is functionally defined as the difference between systemic blood pressure and intracranial pressure.[9] Cerebral perfusion pressure less than 50 torr is known to produce deterioration in neurologic function, presumably as a function of progressive ischemia and accumulation of acid metabolites.[9,35,37] In addition to potentially lowering the systemic blood pressure, the positive intrathoracic pressure produced by PEEP may also impede venous outflow from the cranial vault, leading to increased intracranial pressure.[34,35] PEEP-induced depression of systemic blood pressure, elevation of intracranial pressure, or both, can decrease cerebral perfusion pressure and thus result in neurologic deterioration.[33-37]

There are conflicting reports of the effects of PEEP on intracranial pressure and cerebral perfusion pressure when instituted in head-injured patients.[33-37] Baseline values of intracranial pressure have been reported to increase and even double with institution of PEEP in the presence of intracranial hypertension.[33] However, no consistent correlation between elevations in intracranial pressure and levels of PEEP have been documented using less than 20 cm H_2O of PEEP.[37]

Several factors are no doubt involved in the conflicting findings. Adaptation of systemic circulation to PEEP is variable and often incomplete in severely head-injured patients as a result of volume depletion and alteration of autonomic discharge from the central nervous system.[34] Autoregulation of cerebral vessel diameter and resistance to blood flow normally maintains cerebral blood flow in the face of blood pressure fluctuations.[9] However, in the presence of intracranial hypertension, cerebral compliance is reduced and autoregulatory vessel changes are unable to maintain constant flow.[9] Thus, in the presence of impaired autoregulation cerebral blood flow and perfusion pressure become passively dependent upon systemic blood pressure; generally, the greater the elevation in intracranial pressure the more dependent cerebral perfusion becomes upon systemic pressure.[9] It has been consistently reported that the degree of PEEP-induced increases in intracranial pressure and decreases in cerebral perfusion pressures fluctuates proportionately with the baseline intracranial pressure.[33-37] If cerebral perfusion pressure is maintained above 50 torr, reduction of systemic blood pressure as an isolated factor is probably not the entire basis for neurologic deterioration. PEEP-induced impedance of cerebral venous outflow is also involved and becomes critical in the presence of intracranial hypertension and reduced cerebral compliance. Clearly, the degree of elevation in intracranial pressure prior to institution of PEEP is a critical factor in the patient's ability to tolerate its use. Elevation of the head facilitates cerebral venous outflow and therefore decreases the magnitude of PEEP-induced elevations in intracranial pressure.[35]

Pulmonary compliance is another factor that can affect hemodynamic changes associated with PEEP. The pathological changes associated with neurogenic pulmonary edema and/or adult respiratory distress syndrome decrease lung compliance and therefore are thought to decrease the magnitude of pressure transmission within the thoracic space.[36]

It has been consistently emphasized that the use of PEEP in head-injured patients must be weighed carefully. In situations of severe intracranial hypertension it may be safer to risk the consequences of high-flow oxygen-induced pulmonary damage. If PEEP is deemed necessary, titration of pressures must include consideration of intracranial pressure, intracranial compliance, and systemic blood pressure.[33-35]

CLINICAL IMPLICATIONS

Nursing care of head-injured patients must reflect the fact that respiratory compromise, however subtle, is inherent. Repeated auscultation of lung fields must be performed with aggressive attention to the development of rales. Arterial blood gases need to be analyzed initially and serially, preferably for 3 to 5 days even if initial values are satisfactory. Particular attention must be given to the arterial oxygen tension as a means of detecting development or progression of V/Q mismatch.

Chest x-ray changes characteristically do not occur until pronounced pathology exists, and a "normal" chest x-ray does not preclude the possibility of respiratory compromise. The value of frequent position change cannot be overstated; immobility is a well-known contributor to respiratory dysfunction and atelectasis is extremely likely. The combination of hypoventilation and tendency for gravity-induced increased and inappropriate perfusion of dependent alveoli undoubtedly contribute to preexisting neurogenic pulmonary shunting.[2] Improved matching of ventilation and perfusion through the use of oscillating beds (providing continual lateral rotation) have decreased atelectatic pulmonary changes.[32]

The neurologically compromised individual is vulnerable to many other respiratory problems due to depression of the level of consciousness and basic protective reflexes. Aspiration with subsequent pneumonitis is unfortunately not uncommon and actions to prevent its occurrence should be instituted as routine measures in all individuals unable to protect their own airway. Naso-gastric decompression should be instituted in the absence of bowel tones. Elevation of the head of the bed and prevention of gastric distention aid in prevention of esophageal reflux.

The care of the neurologically compromised patient is complex. Antici-pation of respiratory dysfunction and thorough, serial, pulmonary evaluation are necessary; protective measures must also be instituted. Treatment regimes designed to minimize intracranial pressure will, if effective, have the added benefit of minimizing respiratory complications.

SUMMARY

Neurogenesis and control of respiratory function are complex physiologic processes that involve integration by the central nervous system. With alter-ation of the multiple interactions involved in the dynamic adjustment of res-piration, intracranial pathology is frequently accompanied by respiratory com-plications. These might include varying degrees of altered breathing patterns, ventilation/perfusion mismatch with hypoxemia, neurogenic pulmonary edema, and adult respiratory distress syndrome.

Anticipation of respiratory dysfunction is critical when caring for neuro-logically compromised patients. While abnormalities in the respiratory pattern are generally obvious clinically, ventilation/perfusion mismatches are often subtle and not fully developed upon admission. Satisfactory initial arterial blood gases frequently lead to the assumption that pulmonary follow-up is unnecessary. However, delayed hypoxemia as a function of progressive ven-tilation/perfusion mismatch can be severe and if not corrected can potentially increase existing damage and impede neurologic recovery. Serial pulmonary evaluation, including arterial blood gas analysis, is critical if hypoxemia is to be prevented.

Neurogenic pulmonary edema and adult respiratory distress syndrome associated with central nervous system insult are seemingly rare. Intracranial hypertension is a common denominator in the development of the pathological pulmonary changes associated with both. Treatment, therefore, must include not only correction of the respiratory compromise but control of intracranial pressure as well. Actions such as fluid restriction, diuretics, hyperosmolar agents, supplemental oxygen, and assisted ventilation serve both therapeutic purposes. Positive end-expiratory pressure has also been used but there is controversy over its neurologic effects.

The challenge presented by the neurologically compromised patient is inherently complex. Early detection and treatment of respiratory complications is necessary if optimal return of neurologic function is to be assured. Awareness of the potential complications is the first step but must be followed by aggressive support of pulmonary function.

REFERENCES

1. Slonim NB, Hamilton LH: Respiratory Physiology. 3rd Ed. CV Mosby, St. Louis, 1976.
2. Frost EAM: The physiopathology of respiration in neurosurgical patients. J Neurosurg 50:699–714, 1979.
3. Leitch AG, McLennan JE, Balkenhol S, Loudon RG, McLaurin RL: Mechanisms of hyperventilation in head injury: Case report and review. Neurosurg 5:701–707, 1979.
4. Tenney SM, Ou LC: Ventilatory response of decorticate and decerebrate cats to hypoxia and CO_2. Respir Physiol 29:81–92, 1977.
5. Cohen MI: Respiratory periodicity in the paralyzed, vagotomized cat: Hypocapneic polypnea. Am J Physiol 206:845–854, 1964.
6. Plum F, Posner JB: Diagnosis of stupor and coma. FA Davis, Philadelphia, 1980.
7. Brown HW, Plum F: The neurologic basis of Cheyne-Stokes respiration. Am J Med 30:849–860, 1961.
8. Leitch AG, Balkenhol S, Loudon RG, McLennan JE, McLaurin RL: The reflex hypoxic drive contribution to spontaneous hyperventilation in patients with head injury. Am Rev Respir Dis 119:328, 1979.
9. Shapiro HM: Intracranial hypertension: Therapeutic and anesthetic considerations. Anesthesiology 43:445–471, 1975.
10. Lane DJ, Rout MW, Williamson DH: Mechanism of hyperventilation in acute cerebrovascular accidents. Br Med J 3:9–12, 1971.
11. Dempsey JA, Skatrud JB, Forster HV, Hanson PG, Chosy LW: Is brain ECF (H) an important drive to breath in man? Chest 73:251–253, 1978.
12. Heistad DD, Wheeler RC, Mark AL, Schmid PG, Abboud FM: Effect of adrenergic stimulation on ventilation in man. J Clin Invest 51:1469–1475, 1972.
13. Stone DJ, Keltz H, Sakkar TK, Singzon J: Ventilatory response to adrenergic stimulation and inhibition. J Appl Physiol 34:619–623, 1973.
14. Stanley NN, Kelsen SG, Cherniack NS: Effect of liver failure on ventilatory response to hypoxia in man and the goat. Clin Sci Mol Med 50:25–35, 1976.
15. Bakow ED: Respiratory care of the critically ill patient with head trauma. Crit Care Q 2:81–95, 1979.
16. Pace NL: Fluctuating hypoxemia and pulmonary shunting following fatal head trauma: A case report. Anes Analgesia 56:129–132, 1977.
17. Bricoli A, Truazzi S, Alexandre A, Rizzuto N: Decerebrate rigidity in acute head injury. J Neurosurg 47:680–698, 1977.
18. Adams JH, Mitchell DE, Graham DI, Doyle D: Diffuse brain damage of immediate impact type: Its relationship to "primary brainstem damage" in head injury. Brain 100:489–502, 1977.
19. French BN, Dublin AB: The value of computerized tomography in the management of 1,000 consecutive head injuries. Surg Neurol 7:171–183, 1977.
20. Mitchell DE, Adams JH: Primary focal impact damage to the brainstem in blunt head injuries: Does it exist? Lancet 2:215–218, 1973.

21. Fulton RL, Rayner AVS, Jones C, Gray LA: Analysis of factors leading to post-traumatic pulmonary insufficiency. Ann Thor Surg 25:500–509, 1978.
22. Schumacker PT, Rhodes GR, Newell JC, Dutton RE, Shah DM, Scovill WA, Powers SR: Ventilation-perfusion imbalance after head trauma. Am Rev Respir Dis 119:33–43, 1979.
23. Moss G: Respiratory distress syndrome as a manifestation of primary CNS disturbance. In McLaurin, RL, Ed: Head injuries: Second Chicago symposium on neural trauma. Grune and Stratton, New York, 1976.
24. Frost EAM, Arancibia CU, Schulman K: Pulmonary shunt as a prognostic indicator in head injury. J Neurosurg 50:768–772, 1979.
25. Yen JK, Rhodes GR, Bourke RS, Powers SR, Newell JC, Popp, AJ: Delayed impairment of arterial blood oxygenation in patients with severe head injury: Preliminary report. Surg Neurol 9:323–327, 1978.
26. Katsurada K, Yamada R, Sugimoto T: Respiratory insufficiency in patients with severe head injury. Surg 73:191–199, 1973.
27. Beckman DL, Bean JW, Baslock DR: Neurogenic influence on pulmonary compliance. J Trauma 14:111–115, 1974.
28. Bergen DR, Beckman DL: Pulmonary surface tension and head injury. J Trauma 15:336–338, 1975.
29. Milley JR, Nugent SK, Rogers MC: Neurogenic pulmonary edema in childhood. J Ped 94:706–709, 1979.
30. Cohen HB, Gambill AF, Eggers GWN: Acute pulmonary edema following head injury: Two case reports. Anesth Analg 56:136–139, 1977.
31. Mitchell PH, Mauss H: Intracranial pressure: Fact and fancy. Nursing 76 76:53–57, 1976.
32. Schimmel L, Civetta JM, Kirby RR: A new mechanical method to influence pulmonary perfusion in critically ill patients. Crit Care Med 5:277–278, 1977.
33. Apuzzo MJ, Weiss, MH, Petersons V, Small RB, Kurze T, Heiden JS: Effect of positive end-expiratory pressure ventilation on intracranial pressure in man. J Neurosurg 46:227–232, 1977.
34. Aidinis SJ, Lafferty J, Shapiro HM: Intracranial responses to PEEP. Anesthesiology 45(3):275–286, 1976.
35. Shapiro HM, Marshall LF: Intracranial pressure responses to PEEP in head-injured patients. J Trauma 18(4):254–256, 1978.
36. Huseby JS, Pavlin EG, Butler J: Effect of positive end-expiratory pressure on intracranial pressure in dogs. J Appl Physiol 44(1):25–27, 1978.
37. James HE, Tsueda K, Wright B, Young AB, McCloskey J: The effect of positive end-expiratory pressure (PEEP) ventilation in neurogenic pulmonary oedema. Acta Neurochir 43:275–280, 1978.

5 | Acute Head Injury

Diana L. Nikas
Mary Tolley

Trauma is the third leading cause of death in the first three decades of life and ranks fourth over all age groups.[1] In the United States, more than 100,000 persons die and about 1.5 million are hospitalized annually as the result of trauma.[1] Death from automobile accidents is highest in the 15–24 year old age group, and two thirds of these deaths are the direct result of head trauma.[2] Automobile accidents are the most common cause of head injury, with motorcycle and vehicle-pedestrian accidents, falls, assault, gunshot or stab wounds, and recreational accidents following closely behind.[3] Almost one out of 25 people in the U.S. will suffer head trauma this year.[2]

This chapter will discuss initial care and assessment of the head-injured patient; the specific lesions produced by head trauma; the diagnosis and definitive care of such patients; and protocols for their overall management.

EMERGENCY CARE AND ASSESSMENT

As with any trauma victim, maintenance of adequate respiratory and cardiovascular function is the first priority with head injury.[2,4,5] This includes placing an endotracheal tube in patients who are not fully awake and alert, establishing intravenous routes for fluids and drugs, and inserting an indwelling urinary catheter to assist in the assessment of fluid status and to monitor the effectiveness of diuretic therapy.[6,7] Arterial blood gases should be drawn and supplemental oxygen administered while awaiting results because respiratory insufficiency is a common initial finding in head injury,[7] and causes hypoxemia in a high percentage of patients.[2] Although vomiting occurs in 20% of head-injured patients, it is more common in patients with less severe trauma who

89

are not in deep coma.[8] Emptying the stomach via nasogastric suction precludes vomiting and pulmonary aspiration in these patients.[4,5,9]

Initial assessment of the head trauma victim includes ruling out cervical spine fracture, a commonly associated injury.[2,4,5] The patient will often be admitted wearing a cervical collar, with sand bags appropriately placed by the paramedics. Cervical spine x-rays should be taken and interpreted before moving the patient from the stretcher and before removing the cervical collar and/ or sand bags. Testing for oculocephalic reflexes (doll's eyes) or other movement of the head and neck could result in permanent spinal cord injury if done on a patient with cervical spine instability. A description of the accident and history of the patient must be sought, and frequently the paramedics can be helpful in this regard.

A rapid neurological examination of the patient, repeated at frequent intervals, should include assessment of the level of consciousness, pupillary size and reaction to light, oculocephalic or oculovestibular reflexes, cranial nerve functions, and motor responses. Vital signs provide a great deal of information regarding general status of the patient and may profoundly affect his or her outcome.

Although there is evidence suggesting that glucocorticoids do not influence outcome in severely head-injured patients,[10,11] they are part of the treatment regimen in many institutions.[3,12,13] A loading dose of 10–20 mg of dexamethasone is usually followed by maintenance doses of 4–6 mg every 6 hours, although higher doses have been used.[2,10] Mannitol may be given the severely injured victim who is rapidly deteriorating, in order to gain time to prepare the patient for neurosurgery.[2,4] I.V. doses of 0.25 to 1.0 gm per kg given rapidly have been recommended.[14] An indwelling urinary catheter should be in place when osmotic diuretics are used to prevent bladder damage and to assess the effectiveness of diuresis.

Computerized tomographic (CT) scanning should be done as quickly as possible on any patient whose neurological status is not improving toward normal or who is deteriorating. Skull x-rays should be done if a depressed fracture is suspected. Again, cervical spine injury must be ruled out prior to moving the patient for these studies.

SCALP LACERATIONS

Scalp lacerations are among the most common types of head injury.[15] Because of the extensive vascularity of the scalp and the poor contractility of these vessels when injured, scalp lacerations can result in significant blood loss. With severe lacerations hypovolemia may result.[2,5,15] Direct pressure will usually control bleeding in less severe lacerations, while suturing of the wound may be necessary to control bleeding in more serious injuries. Assessment of scalp lacerations includes careful visual examination and skull x-rays to detect fractures or foreign bodies. Treatment involves shaving the hair around the laceration, irrigating the wound with copious amounts of saline or bacitracin solution, and careful debridement of the wound prior to closure.[2,5,16] Failure to adequately cleanse and debride the wound can lead to subgaleal abscess[2,16] or intracranial infection.

SKULL FRACTURES

Skull fractures fall into one of three major categories: linear, depressed, or basilar. They are further classified as closed if there is no scalp laceration, or open when associated with a scalp laceration or extension of the fracture into the paranasal sinuses or middle ear.[17]

Linear skull fractures constitute approximately 80% of all skull fractures, and 50% of these involve the temporal-parietal bones.[17] Linear skull fractures are the result of elastic deformation of the bone and do not cause displacement of the bone. When an impact of moderate energy and velocity strikes the skull, the area receiving the blow bends inward while the area around it bends outward. The fracture begins at the area of outbending and extends both toward the point of impact and away from it, toward the base of the skull.[17] Normally, linear skull fractures require no specific treatment, except if associated with a scalp laceration or extension of the fracture into the sinuses or middle ear. Then antibiotic therapy is usually required.[5,17] Since the meningeal arteries lie in grooves in the inner table of the skull, fractures that cross one of these branches could lacerate it and lead to an epidural hematoma. The superior sagittal and transverse sinuses are also vulnerable to such injury.[2,5,17,18]

The skull is composed of three layers: the outer table, which lies just under the scalp; the inner table, which lies closest to the brain; and the diploic space, which separates the inner and outer tables. The inner and outer tables are solid bone, while the diploic space is cancellous bone. Depressed skull fractures are those that depress the outer table below the inner table of the adjacent bone.[5] Depressed fractures are classified as open or closed, depending on the presence or absence of scalp lacerations. Open depressed skull fractures require immediate surgery because of the associated risk of infection.[5,17,19] Additionally, bone fragments from comminuted depressed fractures may lacerate brain tissue or become imbedded in a venous sinus, such as the superior sagittal or transverse sinus.[17] Removal of these fragments from the sinuses could lead to hemorrhage,[17] and should be carried out in the operating room.

The clinical presentation of the patient with a depressed skull fracture varies depending on the location and extent of cerebral involvement. Contusion or laceration of brain tissue may cause focal neurological deficits. Depressed fractures involving the frontal bone may result in shattering of the cribiform plate and injury to the frontal poles of the cerebrum.[17] The receptors of the olfactory nerve lie in the nasal mucosa and connect with fibers of the olfactory tract on the inferior surface of the frontal lobe. Injury to the cribiform plate may interrupt these fibers and cause anosmia—loss of the sense of smell.[17] A temporal depressed fracture may injure the seventh (facial) or eighth (acoustic) cranial nerves. The facial nerve passes through a foramen in the temporal bone;

fracture of the bone may lacerate the nerve and lead to facial paralysis on the same side as the injury.[17,20] Disturbances in hearing or equilibrium have been reported in as many as 50% of patients with temporal bone fractures, indicating injury to the acoustic nerve.[17]

The surgical treatment of depressed skull fractures involves removal of all fracture fragments and repair of dural and venous sinus tears.[21] The resultant cranial defect is not repaired by cranioplasty for approximately 6 months because of the immediate postoperative risk of swelling and infection.[21] Although covered by the dura, galea and scalp, the brain underlying the cranial defect must be protected from injury and may require that the patient wear a protective helmet. If the cranial defect is large, care must be taken in the immediate postoperative period to position the patient's head in a way that offers protection to the brain.

A basilar skull fracture extends into either the anterior, middle, or posterior fossae at the base of the skull.[5,20] Presence of these fractures is difficult to confirm on plain skull x-rays, although radiographic findings suggestive of basilar skull fracture include 1) an opaque mastoid sinus; 2) opacity of or an air-fluid level in the sphenoid sinus; 3) pneumocephalus.[2] The clinical signs of an anterior fossa basilar skull fracture include cerebrospinal fluid (CSF) rhinorrhea and bilateral, periorbital ecchymosis. CSF rhinorrhea results from a dural laceration that allows CSF to escape the subarachnoid space and exit via the nasal passages. The patient may complain of nasal congestion or a sweet taste in his mouth.[5,20] The periorbital edema and ecchymosis, sometimes referred to as owl's eyes or racoon's eyes, is caused from bleeding into the orbits as a result of the fracture trauma. Direct eye trauma should be ruled out, however.

Ecchymosis over the mastoid bone, called Battle's sign, and CSF otorrhea are indications of a middle fossa basilar skull fracture.[5] Again, the CSF leak results from a dural tear, but in this case the tympanic membrane also must be ruptured for the CSF to escape via the ear. If the tympanic membrane remains intact, blood or fluid may be evident behind the tympanic membrane on otoscopic examination and the patient may complain of difficulty hearing. An intact tympanic membrane may lead to a CSF rhinorrhea as the fluid follows the path of least resistance through the eustacian tube and nasal passages.[5]

Objectives in the care of patients with basilar skull fractures are to prevent both further tearing of the dura and infection. Factors causing transient rises in intracranial pressure (ICP), i.e., Valsalva's maneuvers, coughing, sneezing, and blowing the nose, could cause further tearing of the dura. Therefore the patient should be instructed to allow the CSF to flow freely and not blow his or her nose, and should be assisted in turning, getting on and off the bedpan, and sliding up in bed. Because there is free communication between the environment and the CSF, contamination has the potential for causing central nervous system infection. Nothing should be put into the nose or ears if a CSF leak is suspected. The CSF should be allowed to flow freely and not be inhibited by packing the nose or ears. Suction catheters, nasogastric tubes, and endotracheal tubes should not be put through the nose. It is policy in our neurosurgical intensive care unit that the dried blood usually found in the ear canal or nares not be cleaned out for fear of contamination. Prophylactic antibiotics are usually given.[5]

Distinguishing between CSF rhinorrhea and the rhinorrhea of the upper respiratory tract requires a high degree of suspicion correlated with the patient's clinical presentation and history. While recommended in some of the most prestigious medical textbooks, Hull and Murrow[22] refuted the use of glucose test strips (commonly used to test the urine for glucose) for differentiating between CSF and mucus; 88% of the patients they studied without dural tears were also found to have glucose in their nasal discharge.

CSF leaks usually stop spontaneously within 7–10 days. Although rare, surgical repair of the dural tear may be indicated for persistent CSF discharge[5] or recurrent meningitis.

CLOSED HEAD INJURY

Closed head injury is generally classified as either concussion or contusion. Definitions of concussion vary, but according to Weiss,[5] patients with cerebral concussion have the following characteristics: 1) some degree, however mild, of neurological dysfunction, although loss of consciousness may not occur; 2) this neurological dysfunction occurs immediately following the trauma, not days later, and 3) complete recovery of neurological function occurs within 6–12 hours, usually sooner. He included headache as a significant neurological symptom, therefore, did not classify head trauma patients with severe headache as suffering from concussion. A focal deficit may result from a concussive blow to a discrete cortical area, e.g., cortical blindness resulting from a blow to the occipital lobe.[5] Retrograde amnesia for the event and for events immediately preceding the trauma is a common finding if the trauma resulted in loss of consciousness.

Disruption of the vascular supply to the brain or nerve fiber damage may be responsible for the partial or complete paralysis of neurological functioning resulting from concussion, although this has not been substantiated by research.[23] Diagnosis is clinically based, as all diagnostic studies are normal. Because seemingly minor head trauma sometimes leads to serious intracranial sequelae, all patients with trauma severe enough to cause loss of consciousness are kept 24 hours for observation in our neurosurgical unit. Patients may be discharged to the care of a responsible adult who has been instructed regarding the signs and symptoms that require rehospitalization.

Postconcussion syndrome, described by Roberts[2] as nonspecific dizziness, visual or equilibrium disturbances, inability to concentrate, memory problems, irritability, and headache that may persist for days to weeks, is a controversial subject. Weiss[5] stated that these symptoms represent psychoneurotic behavior and have no physiological basis. The persistence in the literature of similar description of postconcussion complaints, however, lend support to the existence of such an entity.[23]

Cerebral contusion is a common closed head injury, most frequently caused by motorcycle or automobile accidents.[8] Loss of consciousness in these patients implies widespread cerebral hemisphere or brainstem dysfunction or both.[23] Trauma causes the brain to strike the internal surfaces of the skull and orbital roof, and the sharp edges of the wings of the sphenoid bone at the base of the skull, resulting in bruising and petechial hemorrhages.[8,23] The orbital surfaces of the frontal lobes and the junctions of the frontotemporal lobes are the most vulnerable to this type of injury. The movement of the brain within the cranial vault may be of sufficient force to cause laceration of the tips of the temporal lobes by the sphenoid bones. Depending on the extent of the bruising and the amount of trauma to the vascular walls, an extensive area of necrosis and infarction may occur, leading to further oozing of blood into the injured area. This large damaged area may be mistakenly interpreted as an intracerebral hematoma on CT scan.[8]

Contracoup injuries occur when an area of the brain opposite the site of impact is injured. For example, a blow to the occipital area (coup) may result in contusion to the frontal and/or temporal lobes (contracoup), or trauma to the right parietal lobe may cause contusion to the left temporal lobe.[8] There are, therefore, two areas of injury—the coup and the contracoup.

The clinical presentation of the patient with a cerebral contusion depends on the extent of the damage and the area of brain involved. The symptoms vary from a minimal degree of weakness, sensory or speech disturbance, to complete function loss of areas of the brain. The patient's level of consciousness can range from mild confusion and restlessness, combativeness and wild thrashing about, to coma. Loss of consciousness usually occurs at the time of injury and lasts for varying periods of time. There is significant correlation between the length and depth of coma and the morbidity and mortality of the patient.[24] While there is some experimental evidence suggesting that brainstem reticular activity may be affected, at least temporarily, with blows to the head, clinical observation supports other studies which indicate diffuse cerebral insult as the most likely cause of coma in these patients.[23]

Signs of brainstem contusion involve not only coma but cranial nerve dysfunction and impaired or absent oculocephalic and oculovestibular reflexes. Respiratory and cardiovascular instability are often present. Motor abnormalities can occur with both cerebral and brainstem compression. Both flexor posturing (decorticate) and extensor posturing (decerebrate) are known to occur with massive cerebral injury and do not necessarily indicate primary brainstem insult.[23,25]

Nursing and medical intervention for patients with severe closed head injury is essentially supportive and aimed at controlling intracranial pressure and preventing medical complications, to be discussed later in this paper.

INTRACRANIAL HEMATOMAS

Head injury may be complicated by epidural, subdural, or intracerebral hematomas. These hematomas may occur alone or in combination, and are often associated with some degree of cerebral contusion.[2,5,26] Patterns of neurological dysfunction vary with the type and location of the hematoma, although impairment of consciousness occurs with significant amounts of intracranial bleeding and almost 50% of patients with prolonged unconsciousness have intracranial bleeding.[2] Jennett, et al[24] reported that patients with severe head injury and intracranial hematomas had a poorer outcome than patients without hematomas. This adverse outcome was influenced also by age, with a greater percentage of patients over 40 having hematomas and poorer outcomes.[24]

The incidence of epidural hematomas (EDH) is relatively low, comprising only about 5% of all intracranial hematomas.[2,4,5] Epidural hematomas are usually of arterial origin and most result from injury to the meningeal arteries.[18,27] The meningeal arteries supply the dura and lie in grooves of the inner table of the skull. Skull fractures that lacerate a branch of one of the meningeal arteries are present in a high percentage of cases of EDH.[18] Fractures that cross a major venous channel, such as the superior sagittal or transverse sinus, lead to EDH of venous origin.[18] About 30–40% of patients with EDH classically present with a history of a short period of unconsciousness, followed by a lucid interval lasting minutes to hours. This is followed by irritability, complaints of increasingly severe headaches, and confusion. Without intervention, progressive deterioration of the level of consciousness, ipsilateral pupillary dilatation and loss of light reflex, and contralateral hemiparesis, result from transtentorial herniation. Death is imminent if prompt neurosurgical intervention to remove the hematoma is not carried out.[2,5,18,27,28.] The combination of a skull fracture that crosses a major vascular channel and change in the patient's mental status should immediately alert the clinician to the probability of an EDH.

Prognosis is generally felt to be good in patients with EDH who have surgical intervention prior to neurological decompensation.[27,29] Bruce, et al[4] monitored the intracranial pressure (ICP) of patients with EDH postoperatively and found that 80% had normal ICP and recovered rapidly. The remaining 20% presented with a worse neurological status prior to surgery, had evidence of cerebral edema on CT scan postoperatively, and developed increased ICP that required intensive therapy. Although the recovery of these patients was slower than those without increased ICP, they also made a satisfactory recovery.

Reported mortality figures vary dramatically, however. In one review of 167 patients with EDH, Jamieson and Yelland[35] reported a 15.6% mortality rate, whereas Gallagher and Browder,[28] also reporting on 167 patients in that same year, found a 55% mortality rate. The difference in these mortality figures may be attributed to one or more of the following factors: Gallagher and Browder included 45 patients in their study who had EDH that were not surgically removed; these patients died. All of the patients included in Jamieson and Yelland's study had had surgery. The time period for the Jamieson and Yelland series spanned 11 years (1956–1967), whereas it spanned 25 years (1935–1960) in Gallagher and Browder's study. Improved surgical and medical care may have influenced outcome in the later years of the studies. Lastly, age has been consistently reported to be a significant variable in the outcome of patients with head injury, with morbidity and mortality increasing with age.[3,12,24,27–34] Seventy percent of the patients reported by Gallagher and Browder were between 21 and 60 years of age, whereas only 52% of Jamieson and Yelland's patients fell into that age group. Additionally, more than 44% of Jamieson and Yelland's patients were under 20 years old versus only 20% of Gallagher and

Browder's group. Recent mortality figures of 8%[12] indicate that early surgical intervention of the hematoma and aggressive medical management contribute to good outcome in patients with EDH.

Between 50 and 80% of all EDHs occur in the temporal or temporal-parietal areas.[18,27,28] When they occur outside these areas, the signs and symptoms of transtentorial herniation characteristic of acute EDH do not occur, or have a more insidious onset, and the hematomas are not detected as quickly. In addition, many EDH outside the temporal area are of venous origin and accumulate more slowly, thus allowing time for intracranial compensation to take place. These are referred to as chronic EDH. Clinical signs vary depending on the area of brain involved, but a history of trauma along with patient complaints of persistent headache, nausea, and vomiting should signal the need for CT scanning.[18]

Subdural hematomas (SDH) are the most frequent complication of head injury.[2] They are classified as acute, subacute, or chronic, depending on the rate of progression of symptoms and the appearance of the clot at surgery. Avulsion of the bridging veins that traverse the subdural space is the most likely cause of the collection of blood.[2,35] As venous blood collects in the subdural space, it spreads over the cerebral hemispheres.

Acute SDH are those that present and/or are operated on within 72 hours of injury. The subdural collection of blood is either liquid or clotted.[35,36] Acute SDH may be further classified as simple when not associated with cerebral injury, or complicated when the underlying cerebrum is lacerated or contused.[35] The mortality figures for complicated SDH are reportedly more than twice that for simple SDH.[35] SDH are classified as subacute when the symptoms develop 3–20 days after injury.[35,36] The mortality rate for patients with subacute SDH is almost one third that of acute SDH.[36]

Patients with acute or subacute SDH usually present with marked depression in their level of consciousness. Although they may experience a lucid interval similar to that seen in EDH, in Jamieson and Yellands series of 553 patients, only 13% experienced this phenomenon. Pupillary and motor changes were present in 40% of patients with acute SDH. Patients with associated intracranial injuries or bilateral hematomas had greater neurological deficits and higher morbidity and mortality than those with simple SDH.[4,30,35,36]

The pathogenesis of chronic SDH has not been clearly delineated, although bleeding is less profuse and with time the clot changes character, so that at the end of about two weeks it has the color and consistency of crankcase oil and is frequently surrounded by a membrane.[4,35] Because of the slower accumulation of blood, symptoms of chronic SDH formation often begin insidiously and mimic many other disorders.[2,4,5] In fact, symptoms significant enough to pursue medical attention may be delayed for three weeks or longer. Fogelholm and his colleagues[31] reported a median of 10 weeks between the head trauma and surgery in patients over 60 years of age. Headache and signs of increased ICP were reported more frequently in younger patients, whereas contralateral hemiparesis and other signs of motor impairment were prevalent in the older age groups. These differences were attributed to the decrease in brain weight and increase in space between the brain and skull with increasing age.[31] Hemiparesis ipsilateral to the lesion may be seen in as many as 40% of patients with SDH and is due to compression of the contralateral cerebral peduncle (that area of brain containing the motor fibers) against the edge of the tentorium.[5,26] Pupillary changes tend to remain ipsilateral to the lesion, however, and can be used to localize the lesions.[5]

Chronic SDH are prevalent in older patients and chronic alcoholics,[2,4] and a history of trauma may be absent in as many as 35–50% of cases.[5] Diagnosis is confirmed on CT scan, although chronic SDHs that are isodense to normal brain tissue may be difficult to visualize. SDH gradually liquify and become isodense to brain tissue from days to weeks following trauma.[37] Evidence of an isodense SDH on CT scan may be limited to compression or displacement of the ventricles, although giving the patient an iodine-based contrast agent intravenously may cause the membrane surrounding the SDH to enhance and thus show up on CT scan.[37] If CT scan is unavailable, angiography may be necessary for diagnosis.

The treatment of SDH is somewhat controversial. If the patient is neurologically stable and the CT scan demonstrates a small collection of subdural fluid and little or no shift of the midline cerebral structures, some neurosurgeons elect not to operate because of the increased risk of cerebral edema produced by the operative procedure.[4,25] Chronic SDH are frequently aspirated via burr holes, although Tyson, et al[3] reported that craniectomy may become necessary in the event of repeated accumulation of subdural fluid. Bruce et al[4] recommended a large temporofrontoparietal craniotomy for removal of acute or subacute SDH.

Intracerebral hematomas (ICH) result from hemorrhage into the parenchyma of the brain. They are caused by rupture of aneurysms, gunshot or stab wounds, laceration of brain from depressed skull fracture fragments, as well as trauma.[5,26] ICH may occur immediately after trauma or be delayed for as long as 24 hours.[4,39] Prior to CT scanning, it was difficult to differentiate an ICH from hemorrhagic contusion with edema.[4] Signs and symptoms will vary depending on the area of brain affected and the size of the lesion.[2,5] As in patients with small SDH, surgery may be deferred in patients with ICH who have a stable or improving neurological status. In patients with a large ICH and a deteriorating neurological status, surgery is indicated if the location is amenable to surgical intervention. Monitoring of ICP has been recommended in these patients because as many as 50% will develop increased ICP in the postoperative period.[2]

DIAGNOSIS

Since the advent of computerized tomographic scanning (CT scan), plain skull roentgenograms are of limited value in the diagnosis of head injury. While plain skull x-rays identify the presence of linear and depressed skull fractures and may demonstrate intracranial shifts if the pineal gland is calcified, the CT scan is a more sensitive diagnositic tool. So sensitive is the diagnostic potential of CT scanning, that its ". . . injudicious application may threaten clinical methods of neurological diagnosis."[40] CT scan is fast, safe, and requires few personnel. It has dramatically reduced the need for more invasive diagnostic tests, such as cerebral angiography, or for surgical exploration in cases of cerebral contusion or edema that were mistaken for an ICH.[40] Authors are pointing to the value of correlating serial CT scan with clinical assessments of patients who have severe head injury.[41,42] Sodhu, et al found a poor correlation, however, between CT scan findings and recorded intracranial pressure except when both the CT scan and the ICP were normal.[43]

The CT scanner projects an x-ray through numerous axial sections of brain tissue approximately 13 mm thick. Tissues absorb different amounts of x-ray depending on their density, e.g., bone absorbs more x-ray than CSF. Electronic detectors feed this information into a computer, which gives a value to each of the thousands of readings and forms a matrix that is either printed out in digital form or displayed on an oscilloscope in varying shades of gray. The more dense the tissue, the whiter it appears on the oscilloscope and the higher the digital value. Polaroid or x-ray film is used to record the results for the chart.[40] The scan may be performed first without and then with an iodine-based contrast material, which is given intravenously. Areas of brain in which the blood-brain barrier is disrupted absorb the contrast material, resulting in increased density in that area (described as areas of enhancement).[40] Acute EDH, SDH, and ICH appear as areas of increased density (whiter) on the CT scan, (see Figs. 5.1, 5.2, 5.3) whereas cerebral edema or chronic SDH appear as areas of decreased density (darker) on the scan. Hematomas do not usually enhance with contrast although the membrane that often surrounds a chronic SDH may enhance. The ventricles are clearly outlined on CT scan, allowing for assessment of the size, i.e., compressed or dilated, and the position in relation to midline structures. Contused brain tissue is readily distinguishable from edematous tissue and intracerebral hematomas, a distinction not readily apparent on angiography.[40]

Although rarely necessary for diagnosing head injury in major medical centers, angiography is still the most definitive diagnostic tool where CT scan-

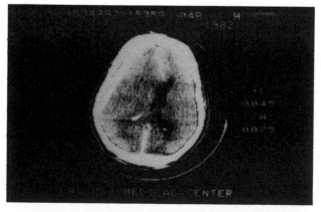

Fig. 5-1.   Left subdural hematoma with a shift from left to right of the lateral ventricles and compression of the left lateral ventricle. There is also a right frontal lobe contusion.

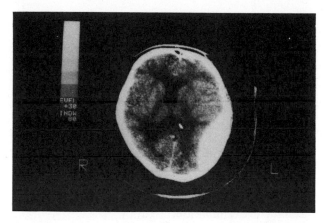

Fig. 5-2. Left parietal-occipital epidural hematoma with a shift of the ventricles from left to right and compression of the posterior horn of the left lateral ventricle.

ning is not available. In addition, angiography remains a very important part in the diagnosis of vascular lesions such as arteriovenous malformations, aneurysms, or highly vascular tumors.[4,40]

Echoencephalography has also been replaced by CT scanning in most hospitals. Its clinical usefulness is generally confined to detecting shifts of normally midline structures. However, if echoencephalography results are correlated with the history and clinical presentation of the patient, they may be valuable in diagnosing head injury when CT scanning is not available. It is not a reliable tool in bilateral lesions or generalized cerebral edema that does not produce a midline shift.[2,5]

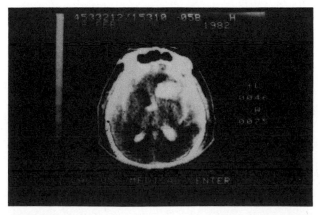

Fig. 5-3. Right frontal intracerebral hematoma with intraventricular hemmorhage.

PROTOCOL FOR MANAGEMENT

The Glasgow Coma Scale evaluates eye opening, motor responses, and verbal responses of the patient (Table 5-1). This scale was devised to predict the outcome of severely head-injured patients, i.e., patients in coma for six hours or longer, in order to assist the clinician in making therapeutic judgments.[24,32-34] The severely head-injured patient in deep coma remains the most difficult to make therapeutic decisions for. Morbidity and mortality figures have remained unremittingly high in these cases.[24] Proper application of the Glasgow Coma Scale for severely head-injured patients seems an appropriate method of attempting to improve those morbidity and mortality figures.[34]

It must be emphasized that the Glasgow Coma Scale is not meant to replace a complete neurological examination. Examination of the fundi of the eyes, pupillary reflexes, cranial nerves, tendon reflexes, and vital signs, as well as detailed descriptions of the level of consciousness, are still necessary.

Management of head-injured patients involves three major aspects 1) surgical removal of mass lesions; 2) control of intracranial pressure; and 3) prevention of complications. The importance or rapid diagnosis and removal of intracranial hematomas has been consistently emphasized[2,3,5,13,25,27-30,34,35,42,44-46] and Rose, et al[19] reported that delay in surgical removal of hematomas was the leading intracranial cause of death in patients with head injury who had talked after injury only to die later. The causes of delay included failure to recognize the significance of the degree and rate of the patients neurological deterioration, or attributing this deterioration to alcoholic intoxication or other neurological pathology. The importance of surgical intervention was further illustrated by a report that failure to recognize and/or remove the epidural hematoma in 45 patients led to their demise.[28]

In patients with mass lesions and associated cerebral injury, the morbidity and mortality figures have been higher than in head-injured patients without mass lesions.[12,25,28] Bowers and Marshall,[3] however, reported no significant difference in outcome for patients with or without mass lesions and attributed this improvement in morbidity and mortality to rapid transport of patients to a skilled medical facility, availability of CT scanning, and aggressive therapy that included early surgical removal of mass lesions.

The need for and value of controlling intracranial hypertension has been the source of increasing research in recent years. With the widespread use of intracranial pressure monitoring to assess and monitor intracranial dynamics, has come the hope of decreasing the previously high mortality figures of 50% or more reported in severely head-injured patients.[24,32,33] Researchers in three medical centers in the United States have challenged these mortality figures by instituting specific treatment protocols for severely head-injured patients.[3,12,13,29,45] The resulting mortality figures from these three groups were reported as 29%,[13] 30%[12] and 36%,[3] a significant improvement over previously reported figures.

Primary injury to the brain is a variable that cannot be controlled. There has been fear that, although mortality figures may improve, the incidence of

TABLE 5-1. Glasgow Coma Scale[a]

Eyes	Open	Spontaneously	**4**
		To verbal command	**3**
		To pain	**2**
	No Response		**1**
Best motor response	To verbal command	Obeys	**6**
	To painful stimulus* (Apply pressure to nailbeds)	Localizes pain	**5**
		Flexion-withdrawal	**4**
		Flexion-abnormal (Decorticate rigidity)	**3**
		Extension (Decerebrate rigidity)	**2**
		No response	**1**
Best verbal response (Arouse patient with painful stimulus if necessary)		Oriented and converses	**5**
		Disoriented and converses	**4**
		Inappropriate words	**3**
		Incomprehensible sounds	**2**
		No response	**1**
Total			**3-15**

[a] The Glasgow Coma Scale, which is based upon eye opening, verbal and motor responses, is a practical means of monitoring changes in level of consciousness. If each response on the scale is given a number (high for normal and low for impaired responses), the responsiveness of the patient can be expressed by summation of the figures. The lowest score is 3; the highest is 15. Features of coma during the first week after severe head injury have been analyzed in 700 patients. Although each step on each part of the scale may not be of equal significance, the method is useful in comparing the overall responsiveness of one patient with another or one series of patients with another. Based of observations of the 700 patients, all combinations that summed seven or less were defined as coma. (From Jennett B, Teasdale G: Aspects of coma after severe head injury. Lancet April 23: pp. 878–881, 1977.)

patients remaining in vegetative or severely disabled states also would increase and thereby not represent true improvement at all.[3,12,24,25,29,32–34] However, an incidence of 10–13% of severely disabled or vegetative survivors was reported by the three previously mentioned groups,[3,12,13] a decrease over earlier reports. These researchers independently concluded that ICP monitoring, which guided the treatment of intracranial hypertension, played a vital role in the improved outcome of their patients with severe head injury.[3,12,13] The protocols for controlling intracranial hypertension included hyperventilation, control of blood pressure, maintenance of normothermia, and pharmacologic agents such as glucocorticoids, diuretic and barbiturate therapy.

Prevention of medical complications has been of major concern in the care of head-injured patients. For this reason, most authors stress the importance of adequate oxygenation, ventilation, and circulation in the care of these critically ill patients. Other complications that require careful attention include control of seizure activity, prevention of hyperthermia, and prevention of fluid and electrolyte problems.

Acute respiratory insufficiency is a common initial finding in head injury[7] and causes hypoxemia in a high percentage of patients.[2] Hypoxia causes profound cellular swelling (cytotoxic cerebral edema),[47,48,52] and vasodilatation that leads to vascular congestion.[2,47] It thus contributes to increased ICP and is associated with worsening of the patients clinical status.[2,6,7] In fact, hypoxia has been reported as a leading extracranial cause of avoidable death in head-injured patients.[19] There is also abundant evidence that intracerebral lactic acidosis, caused by local hypoxia and/or ischemia, occurs after brain injury[6] and further compromises cerebral functioning by altering the pH of the tissues. For these reasons, endotracheal intubation and assisted mechanical ventilation with supplemental oxygen is considered a priority in the care of head-injured patients.[6,7,9] To maximize oxygen diffusion into injured brain tissue, Judson[7] suggested that 100% oxygen be administered for 24 hours after injury, followed by an inspired oxygen sufficient to maintain an arterial oxygen tension higher than normal.

Acute respiratory insufficiency also causes hypercarbia which, along with hypoxia, contributes to cerebral vasodilatation, increased cerebral blood flow, and increased ICP.[6,7,46,49] This increase in ICP could worsen intracranial bleeding[2] and cause ischemia and infarction.[9] Hyperventilation to a $PaCO_2$ of 25–30 mm Hg has been cited as a critical aspect of the care of head-injured patients because it leads to vasoconstriction, thereby reducing cerebral blood volume and ICP.[2–4,6,7,24,45,46] It may also improve regional distribution of cerebral blood flow through damaged areas of the brain.[6,7] Hyperventilation may contribute to normalization of the pH of the CSF and cerebral tissues, which may contribute to improvement in the patient's clinical status.[6]

Control of blood pressure is critical in the overall management of patients with severe head injury. Hypotension may result from hemorrhage of associated injuries such as severe scalp lacerations, chest or abdominal trauma, or fractured extremities.[2,5,15] Hypotension compromises cerebral perfusion pressure and should be treated with appropriate blood and fluid replacement.[2,50] Shock contributes to poor outcome and death in severely head-injured patients.[3,19] Shock due to brain injury alone was reported as rare, was always accompanied by signs of brainstem involvement, and has been associated with a 90% mortality.[50] It must be remembered that intracranial hemorrhage cannot be of sufficient quantity to lead to hypovolemia in the adult, so other causes must be vigorously sought in patients presenting with hypotension. Hypertension contributes to increased intracranial pressure by overcoming autoregulation and increasing cerebral blood flow and hydrostatic pressure.[46] Methods of controlling arterial hypertension include nitroprusside, trimethophan and barbiturates.[12,13,45]

Seizures increase the metabolic needs of the brain and cause increased cerebral blood flow, contributing to increased ICP. The incidence of posttraumatic seizures is difficult to determine, but is estimated to be between 30 and 60% in patients with severe head injury.[51] Seizure activity can progress to status epilepticus and contributes to death if not aggressively treated;[19] anticonvulsants are therefore part of the therapeutic regimen in many medical centers.[2,5,12,51] A loading dose of one gm of phenytoin intravenously followed by maintenance of therapeutic blood levels (20–40 mcg/ml) is recommended.[51]

Hyperthermia also increases the metabolic needs of the brain, and is thus vigorously combated in the head-injured patient. While hypothermia decreases cerebral metabolic needs and should theoretically offer protection for the injured brain, it is infrequently utilized as a therapeutic intervention and then only in conjunction with other forms of therapy for control of intracranial hypertension. Normothermia has been recommended as part of the protocol for the management of head injury.[12,45]

The fluid and electrolyte abnormalities most often encountered in head-injured patients are water and sodium imbalances. These imbalances may result from injury to the hypothalamus or pituitary gland, or occur secondarily to fluid and drug therapy. Fluids are generally restricted in head-injured patients, and if the restriction is severe, may lead to dehydration and hypovolemia. In addition, many drugs for the control of intracranial pressure, such as osmotic and loop diuretics, glucocorticoids, and barbiturates, may contribute to water and sodium imbalances. Both diabetes insipidus and syndrome of inappropriate secretion of antidiuretic hormone result in fluid and electrolyte changes which may become severe if not monitored closely and treated promptly.[53]

In summary, most protocols for the management of patients with severe head injury include 1) rapid transport to a trauma center; 2) intubation and mechanical ventilation to insure oxygenation and hyperventilation; 3) early detection and surgical removal of intracranial mass lesions; 4) control of intracranial hypertension, including the use of intracranial pressure monitoring; 5) prevention of seizure activity; 6) control of body temperature; and 7) treatment of fluid and electrolyte imbalances.

REFERENCES

1. Wilson RF: Trauma. Critical care state of the art. Proceedings Society of Critical Care Medicine, Anaheim, 1980.
2. Roberts JR: Pathosphysiology, diagnosis and treatment of head trauma. Topics in Em Med 1:41–62, 1979.
3. Bowers SA, Marshall LF: Outcome in 200 consecutive cases of severe head injury treated in San Diego County: A prospective analysis. Neurosurgery 6:237–242, 1980.
4. Bruce DA, Gennarelli TA, Langfitt TW: Resuscitation from coma due to head injury. Crit Care Med 6:254–269, 1978.
5. Weiss MH: Axioms on the management of head injury. Hosp Med 11:94–110, 1975.

6. Gorgon E: Nonoperative treatment of acute head injuries: The Korolinska Experience. Int Anesthesiol Clin 17:181–199, 1979.

7. Judson JA: Nonoperative treatment of severe head injuries: The Auckland Experience. Int Anesthesiol Clin 17:153–180, 1979.

8. Thomas LM, Gurdjion ES: Cerebral contusion in closed head injury and nonoperative management of head injury. In: Youmans JR (Ed): Neurologic Surgery. WB Saunders, Philadelphia, 1973.

9. Caronna JJ and Simon RP: The comatose patient: A diagnostic approach and treatment. Int Anesthesiol Clin 17:3–18, 1979.

10. Cooper PR, Moody S, Clark W, et al: Dexamethasone and severe head injury: A prospective double blind study. J Neurosurg 51:307–316, 1979.

11. Gudeman SK, Miller JD, Becker DP: Failure of high dose steroid therapy to influence intracranial pressure in patients with severe head injury. J Neurosurg 51:301–306, 1979.

12. Becker DP, Miller JD, Ward D, et al: The outcome from severe head injury with early diagnosis and intensive management. J Neurosurg 47:491–502, 1977.

13. Levin AB, Duff TA, Javid MJ: Treatment of increased intracranial pressure: A comparison of different hyperosmotic agents and the use of thiopental. Neurosurg 5:570–574, 1979.

14. Marshall LF, Smith RW, Rauscher LA, et al: Mannitol dose requirements in brain injured patients. J Neurosurg 48:169–172, 1978.

15. Dingman RO: Injuries to the scalp. In: Youmans JR: Neurological Surgery. WB Saunders, Philadelphia, 1973.

16. Goodman SJ, Cohen L, Chow AW: Subgaleal abscess: A preventable complication of scalp trauma. West J Med 127:169–172, 1977.

17. Thomas LM, Hodgsen VR, Gurdjion S: Skull fractures and management of open head injury. In: Youmans JR (Ed): Neurologic Surgery. WB Saunders, Philadelphia, 1973.

18. Hirsh LF: Chronic epidural hematomas. Neurosurgery 6:508–512, 1980.

19. Rose J, Valtonen S, Jennett B: Avoidable factors contributing to death after head injury. Brit J Med 2:615–618, 1977.

20. Bales R: Facial, auditory and vestibular nerve injuries associated with basilar skull fractures. In: Youmans JR (Ed): Neurologic Surgery. WB Saunders, Philadelphia, 1973.

21. Timmins RL: Cranial defects and their repair. In: Youmans JR (Ed): Neurologic Surgery. WB Saunders, Philadelphia, 1973.

22. Hull HF, Murrow G: Gluorrhea revisited: Prolonged promulgation of another plastic pearl. JAMA 234:1052–1053, 1975.

23. Plum F, Posner JB: The Diagnosis of Stupor and Coma. FA Davis, Philadelphia, 1980.

24. Jennett B, Teasdale G, Braakman R, et al: Prognosis of patients with severe head injury. Neurosurgery 4:282–289, 1979.

25. Bricolo A, Turazzi S, Feriotti G: Prolonged traumatic unconsciousness. J Neurosurg 52:625–634, 1980.

26. Thomas LM, Gurdjion ES: Intracranial hematomas of traumatic origin. In: Youmans JR (Ed): Neurologic Surgery. WB Saunders, Philadelphia, 1973.

27. Jamieson KG, Yelland JDN: Extradural hematoma. Experience with 167 patients. J Neurosurg 29:13–23, 1968.

28. Gallagher JP, Browder EJ: Extradural hematoma. J Neurosurg 29:1–12, 1968.

29. Miller JD, Becker DP, Ward JD, et al: Significance of intracranial hypertension in severe head injury. J Neurosurg 47:503–516, 1977.
30. Fell DA, Fitzgerald S, Moiel RH, et al: Acute subdural hematomas: Review of 144 cases. J Neurosurg 42:37–42, 1975.
31. Fogelholm R, Heiskonen O, Waltimo O: Chronic subdural hematomas in adults: Influence of patient's age on symptoms, signs and thickness of hematoma. J Neurosurg 42:43–46, 1975.
32. Jennett B: Severe head injury: Prediction for outcome as a basis for management decisions. Int Anesthesiol Clin 17:133–152, 1979.
33. Jennett B, Teasdale G, Braakman R, et al: Predicting outcome in individual patients after severe head injury. Lancet 1:1031–1034, 1976.
34. Langitt TW: Measuring the outcome from head injuries. J Neurosurg 48:673–678, 1978.
35. Jamieson KG, Yelland JDN: Surgically treated traumatic subdural hematomas. J Neurosurg 37:137–149, 1972.
36. Rosenorn J, Gjerris F: Long-term follow-up of patients with acute and subacute subdural hematomas. J Neurosurg 48:345–349, 1978.
37. Shields CB, Sites TB, Garretson HD: Isodense subdural hematoma presenting with paraparesis. J Neurosurg 52:712–714, 1980.
38. Tyson G, Strachan WE, Newman P, et al: The role of cranioectomy in the treatment of chronic subdural hematomas. J Neurosurg 52:776–781, 1980.
39. Brown FD, Mullon S, Duda EE: Delayed traumatic intracerebral hematoma: Report of 3 cases. J Neurosurg 48:1019–1022, 1978.
40. Marshall LF, Shapiro HM: Examination by computerized axial tomography. Int Anesthesiol Clin 17:391–411, 1979.
41. Clifton GL, Grossman RG, Makela ME, et al: Neurological course and correlated computerized tomography findings after severe closed head injury. J Neurosurg 52:611–624, 1980.
42. Sweet RC, Miller JD, Lipper M, et al: Significance of bilateral abnormalities in the CT scan in patients with head injury. Neurosurgery 3:16–21, 1979.
43. Sodhu VK, Sompron J, Haar FL, et al: Correlation between computed tomography and intracranial pressure monitoring in acute head trauma patients. Radiology 133:507–509, 1979.
44. Bricolo A, Turazzi S, Alexandre A, Rizzuto N: Decerebrate rigidity in acute head injury. J Neurosurg 47:680–698, 1977.
45. Marshall LF, Smith RW, Shapiro HM: The outcome with aggressive treatment in severe head injuries. Part 1: The significance of intracranial pressure monitoring. J Neurosurg 50:20–25, 1979.
46. Miller JD, Sullivan HG: Severe intracranial hypertension. Int Anesthesiol Clin 17:19–75, 1979.
47. Fishman RA: Brain edema. N Engl J Med 293:706–711, 1975.
48. Ignelzi RJ: Cerebral edema: Present perspectives. Neurosurgery 4:338–342, 1979.
49. Leitch AG, McLennean JE, Balkenhol S, et al: Mechanisms of hyperventilation in head injury: Case report and review. Neurosurgery 5:701–707, 1979.
50. Youmans JR: Causes of shock with head injury. J Trauma 4:204–209, 1964.
51. Wohns RNW, Wyler AR: Prophylactic phenytoin in severe head injuries. J Neurosurg 51:507–509, 1979.
52. Trubuhovich RV: Acute brain swelling. Int Anesthesiol Clin 17:77–131, 1979.
53. Nikas DL: Fluid resuscitation of the head-injured patient. In Ellerbe S, Ed: Con-

temporary Issues in Critical Care Nursing. Vol. 1: Churchill Livingstone, New York, 1981.

SUGGESTED READINGS

Jennett B, Teasdale G: Management of Head Injury. FA Davis, Philadelphia, 1981.

6 | Acute Spinal Cord Injuries: Care and Complications

Diana L. Nikas

Acute spinal cord injury occurs most commonly in young active adults as the result of trauma.[1] All systems of the body can be affected by this injury, the severity of symptoms varying with the level and extent of injury. Emphasis in this chapter will be on those effects of acute spinal cord injury that may be manifested during the first 3 to 10 days after injury, either as a result of or related to the stage of spinal shock. They include effects on the cardiovascular, respiratory, gastrointestinal, and genitourinary systems with reference to how these systems are affected by spinal shock; fluid and electrolyte problems encountered by these patients and the alteration producing the disorder; implications for nursing care; theories related to the pathophysiology of spinal cord injury; current concepts in the early treatment of injury will be correlated to theories related to the pathogenesis of spinal cord injury.

SPINAL SHOCK

The spinal cord contains afferent tracts that receive sensory information from the periphery and conduct it to the brain, and efferent tracts that control motor responses and mediate many autonomic functions. In spite of considerable protection afforded the spinal cord, its function can be interrupted by disruption of the vertebrae or blood flow. Traumatic lesions of the spinal cord are often classified as complete when there is interruption of all afferent and efferent nerve tracts below the level of injury, or incomplete when some tracts are spared.

Sudden transection of the spinal cord leads to spinal shock, a state of transient reflex depression below the level of injury. The pathophysiologic cause of spinal shock, based on the work of Sherrington in 1897, is the "... sudden withdrawal of [the] predominantly facilitory influence of descending supraspinal tracts from higher centers, resulting in a disruption of transmission at the synapse and thus rendering the process of conduction impossible or difficult."[2] Research in recent years has revealed additional factors involved in the mechanism of spinal shock: persistent inhibition from below the lesion acting on extensor reflexes and axonal degeneration of neurons, this degeneration being more severe when the axon is severed near the cell body.[3] The intensity of spinal shock varies with the level of injury, and some distal reflexes, both cutaneous and tendon, may be retained, although diminished, in cervical transection or may be lost later in spinal shock.[2] The anal reflex may never be lost, although Guttmann pointed out that this retained reflex activity in no way indicates that the lesion is incomplete. The duration of spinal shock varies considerably in man, reflex activity reappearing anywhere from a few days to 6 weeks or even months after injury; return may be delayed by infection.[2]

Reflex depression occurs predominantly caudal to the lesion, with reflexes closer to the lesion being more severely affected and for a greater period of time. Reflex depression can also occur rostral to the lesion and represents a concussional effect of cord transection with resultant edema.[2,4,5] This more rostral impairment is transient, and function usually returns within a few days. As a result of areflexia, the paralysis of spinal shock is flaccid in nature, even though the lesion is of an upper motor neuron (suprasegmental type). Once spinal shock has subsided and reflex function returns, the spasticity characteristic of upper motor neuron lesions is manifest.[1]

Reflex return generally occurs in a rostral direction, with anal and bulbocavernosus reflexes and response to plantar stimulation occurring earlier. There is, however, a great deal of variability of reflex return after spinal shock.[6] If there is a longitudinal lesion of the spinal cord in addition to the transverse lesion, reflexes for the muscle groups innervated by those spinal cord segments (and perhaps for muscles below the level of the lesion) may never return; i.e., they exhibit a lower motor neuron (segmental) type of paralysis. Again, septic and toxic conditions may alter reflex return.[6]

Sensory modalities mediated by the posterior columns (position and vibratory sense and touch), anterolateral spinothalamic tracts (pain and temperature senation), and ventrodorsal spinocerebellar tract (proprioception, touch, and pressure sensation), are lost below the level of the lesion during spinal shock. Initially there is a distinct line of sensory demarcation that later becomes dissociated as spinal segments "... assume their compensatory overlapping of sensory function."[6] Phantom sensations, as well as burning and tingling below the level of the lesion, may be manifested.[6]

Emergency Care

All patients with multiple trauma, especially those who have sustained head trauma, should be treated as if they have a cervical spine injury until proven otherwise by radiographic examination.[7] The spinal cord-injured victim requires immediate attention in three areas: immobilization of the head and neck, and restoration and maintenance of respiratory and cardiovascular functions. Optimal care requires early detailed assessment and rapid transport to a facility where the personnel are skilled in the care of spinal cord-injured patients.

Immobilization of the victim is usually accomplished by paramedics at the scene with either a spine board or cervical collar or both; these should be applied before moving the victim. The head should be maintained in a neutral position and slight traction applied to the neck during transfer.[8,9] The victim should be placed on a hard, flat surface with sandbags on either side of his head, and she/he should be instructed not to sit up or turn his/her head. Sandbags serve to remind the patient to remain immobile and alert health care personnel that the patient has a potentially unstable spine. The patient should be kept on the stretcher he arrives on until the final decision is made regarding the type of bed on which to place him.

In addition to immobilization, immediate administration of glucocorticoids in the field has been advocated[10,11] although their efficacy has been questioned.[7]

Increasing emphasis is being placed on the immediate transport of the victim, by the fastest and safest method possible, to a facility skilled in the care and treatment of spinal cord-injured patients, i.e., a spinal cord injury center.[7,9,13] Transport often requires specially designed ambulances or aircraft, and attendance of highly trained nurses and physicians. Therapies currently being investigated as being potentially beneficial in spinal cord trauma have been shown to be most effective if instituted within 4 hours of the trauma, further emphasizing the need for rapid safe transport. Rapid transport to a skilled facility has also proven effective in reducing the number of spinal cord-injured patients who are admitted with complete lesions.[13]

Acceptable cervical spine x-rays must include all seven cervical vertebrae and anterior-posterior as well as lateral views should be obtained. The neurosurgeon should assist in obtaining views other than lateral to ensure adequate protection to the spine during the maneuver.[14]

The need for respiratory assistance must be carefully evaluated, since respiratory failure is a primary cause of death in acute cervical injury.[7] Endotracheal intubation via the nasal route to avoid hyperextention of the neck will facilitate the respiratory care of the patient. Because patients with complete transections of the spinal cord at the high thoracic or low cervical level will have only diaphragmatic function, arterial blood gases should be monitored to detect inadequate ventilation or oxygenation. Measurement of vital capacity and tidal volume will aid in assessing the patient's ability to maintain ventilation unassisted, and indicate whether he will be able to cough and deep breathe and thus prevent atelectasis. If the patient has a respiratory arrest prior to intubation, the American Heart Association Standards for Basic Life Support recommend that a modified jaw-thrust method be used to establish an airway.

Cervical or high thoracic cord lesions that interrupt the sympathetic outflow result in hypotension and can be severe in some patients.[8] Hypotension is usually adequately treated with fluid replacement although the patient must be monitored carefully to avoid volume overload. Associated injuries must be sought for their role in the production of hypotension. Bradycardia often accompanies hypotension due to sympathetic ablation, and does not allow the body to compensate for the reduced cardiac output. These issues become critical when other injuries are present.

Neurological assessment of the patient includes evaluation of motor and sensory function. Baseline assessment should be done immediately and the patient reassessed at frequent intervals. Guttmann[14] emphasized both the medical and legal importance of complete detailed descriptions of the patient's status, including details of the accident. Any muscle movement must be documented, along with a description of reflexes that are lost or retained. The victim should be evaluated for signs of cerebral dysfunction as the result of head trauma.

Assessment of the patient includes special attention to the following: voluntary motor control (corticospinal tracts), i.e., what the patient can move; position and vibratory sense (posterior columns); pain and temperature sensation (anterolateral spinothalamic tracts). The objective of motor assessment is to test the function of all major muscle groups and to evaluate their relative strength. The patient is asked to flex, extend, abduct, and adduct his or her upper and lower extremities to assess the function of the involved muscle groups (Table 6-1). Flexion and extension of the wrist should not be overlooked. The function of the tracts of the posterior columns (fasciculus gracilis and fasciculus cuneatus) is assessed by testing either position or vibratory sense, because testing one will indicate the functioning of the other; both should be tested if results are ambiguous. Position sense is tested by asking the patient to close his eyes and identify if a finger or toe is moved away from or toward

Table 6-1. Muscle Testing for Motor Strength

Motor Action	Muscle Tested	Spinal Cord Segment
Abduction of arm	Deltoid	C–5
Flexion of forearm	Biceps	C–6
Extension of forearm	Triceps	C–7
Flexion of digits 2, 3, 4, & 5	Flexor digitorum superficialis and profundus	C8
Opposition of metacarpal of the thumb	Opponens pollicis	T1
Hip flexion	Iliopsoas	L1–2
Knee extension	Quadriceps femoris	L3
Dorsiflexion of foot	Tibialis anterior	L4
Dorsiflexion of big toe	Extensor hallucis longus	L5
Plantar flexion of foot and big toes	Gastrocnemius flexor hallucis longus	S1–2

Table 6-2. Tendon and Cutaneous Reflex Testing

Deep Tendon Reflexes	Spinal Cord Segment
Biceps	C5–6
Brachioradialis	C5–6
Triceps	C7–8
Finger flexion	C7–T1
Quadriceps (patellar)	L2–4
Achilles (ankle jerk)	L5–S1–3

Superficial Reflexes	Spinal Cord Segment
Upper abdominal*	T7–9
Lower abdominal*	T11–12
Cremasteric*	L1–2
Plantar†	S1–2

* These reflexes are absent in upper motor neuron lesions.

† The Babinski sign is the result of upper motor neuron lesions in response to plantar stimulation.

the head. Vibratory sense is assessed by applying a tuning fork to bony prominences and asking the patient to identify whether or not he feels vibration. The functions of the anterolateral spinothalamic tracts are also assessed by testing one of the major functions. Pain perception is most commonly tested by having the patient close his eyes and identify when he feels a pin prick. Both sides of the body are tested and the sensory level is described on each side in relation to the distance from anatomical landmarks: iliac crest, umbilicus, nipples, or clavicle. Care must be taken not to pierce or scratch the skin with the pin. Test tubes of hot and cold water can be used to assess temperature perception. Tendon and cutaneous reflexes should also be tested and recorded frequently (Table 6-2).

Cardiovascular Effects

The effects of spinal shock on the cardiovascular system are mainly due to loss of sympathetic outflow caused by spinal cord transection above the fifth thoracic spinal segment and is more pronounced in cervical lesions.[15,16,17] The sympathetic nervous system supplies all vessels of the body and maintains vasomotor tone via the sympathetic vasoconstrictor fibers which are stimulated by continuous tonic firing of the vasomotor centers in the brainstem. When impulses from higher brain centers are inhibited, such as by spinal cord transection, vasoconstrictor tone is lost throughout the body and vasodilatation and hypotension result.[18,19] The decreased venous return resulting from the lack of sympathetic tone is additionally complicated by failure of the pumping action of the muscles on the vessels due to paralysis. The hypotension thus produced is not particularly responsive to vasopressors, and increased infusion of fluids in an effort to maintain the blood pressure may lead to pulmonary complications.[16] Although the hypotension is usually self-limiting and does not produce significant perfusion problems if the patient is kept supine,[6] on occasion it may be profound and threaten the perfusion of the kidneys and spinal cord. This is especially dangerous when there are associated injuries complicated by blood loss. The effects of hemorrhage are compounded by lack of compensatory sympathetic vasoconstriction due to sympathetic blockade.[6,7,30,31] Owing to the cardiovascular instability of these patients, surgical complications are more prevalent in the first month after injury.[22] Vasomotor response returns over a period of months in most patients.[18]

The effects of blood pressure alterations on the pathogenesis of spinal cord lesions were studied by Rawe, Lee, and Perot.[23] They demonstrated that hypertension resulted in increased hemorrhage and edema formation in the gray and white matter following experimentally produced spinal cord lesions in cats. Hypotension led to decreased hemorrhage and edema. They concluded that these changes were probably the result of impaired autoregulation of the spinal cord vasculature. Because of impaired autoregulation, hypotension could lead to ischemia of the spinal cord and maintenance of normotension was considered optimal in the care of spinal cord-injured patients.[23] Others have found no changes in the development of hemorrhagic necrosis in the spinal cord with changes in blood pressure.[24]

Fluid replacement for these patients should be carried out cautiously and hemodynamic monitoring used as a guideline for therapy. Urine output should be measured continuously.[7]

Venous Thrombosis and Pulmonary Embolus. Although the hypotension produced by spinal shock is generally not thought to comprise circulation significantly, other complications can occur as the result of decreased sympathetic tone. Decreased rate of blood flow contributes to increased risk of thrombosis of the legs and pelvis.[6,16,25,26] In addition, flaccid paralysis of the intercostal and abdominal muscles in the acute stages of injury contributes to venous stasis as a result of the decrease in negative intrathoracic pressure which normally aids venous return to the heart.[6] Thrombokinase, an enzyme that aids clotting, may also be released in traumatic injury.[6]

Pulmonary embolus can result from venous thrombosis, and patients with cervical injuries are particularly at risk. Although the incidence of thrombosis in patients with cervical injuries is not a great deal higher than in patients with injuries in other parts of the spinal cord, pulmonary embolus is more often fatal to these patients because of their compromised respiratory function and inadequate respiratory reserve.[27–30] Pulmonary embolus has been cited as a leading cause of death (i.e., death within 2 months of injury) by a number of authors.[6,25,31,32]

An incidence of venous thrombosis of 16–17%, with 8–10% resulting in pulmonary embolus, has been reported.[28,30] There was a higher incidence of thrombosis in complete lesions (22%) compared with incomplete lesions (14%).[27] Venous thrombosis most commonly occurred 2 to 3 weeks after injury. Pulmonary embolus usually occurred coincident with the diagnosis of venous thrombosis, often without warning, and had a 2.5–8% mortality.[28,30] Clinical observation for the signs and symptoms of thrombosis is of no value in pelvic thrombi[31] and recent research has revealed that it is often inadequate in detecting thrombosis in lower extremities.[32] Fifty percent of patients with deep vein thrombosis, as diagnosed by the ^{125}I-fibrinogen test, had no signs or symptoms, and when thrombus formation did occur, it began within 5 days after an operative procedure.[32]

Prophylactic anticoagulant therapy has been recommended for the prevention of venous thrombus formation and pulmonary emboli.[6,16,26,31] Silver[31] reported a 5% incidence of venous thrombosis in spinal cord-injured patients who were treated with prophylactic anticoagulation versus 25% without anticoagulation. He pointed out that the diagnosis of pulmonary embolus in a quadraplegic patient was difficult owing to their inability to cough (i.e., hemoptysis will not be apparent) and anesthesia of the chest wall. Clinical signs of sudden onset of respiratory distress and abnormalities of arterial blood gases should suggest further investigation for pulmonary embolus in these patients. Casas et al.[26] reported that in 18 spinal cord-injured patients who received 5000–7000 IU (international units) heparin every 12 hours (no route reported), no venous thrombosis, as diagnosed by leg measurement, or pulmonary embolus occurred. Watson[29] treated 82 spinal cord-injured patients with heparin 5000 units subcutaneously twice a day for 1 month, followed by warfarin therapy for 2 months. There was a 6% incidence of venous thrombosis with a 6% incidence of pulmonary embolus in patients with complete lesions and 0% in patients with incomplete lesions. There were no deaths from pulmonary embolus and no complications of anticoagulant therapy. Frankel and Mathias[25] recommended starting anticoagulant therapy 5 days post injury if there were no contraindications (head trauma, internal bleeding, or history of ulcers), using oral anticoagulants sufficient to keep the prothrombin time two to three times the control. They maintained this therapy for 8 weeks or longer and stated that it provided "absolute protection against fatal pulmonary embolism." They further stated that they had found no other effective prophylaxis against pulmonary emboli. Salzman[34] stated that in light of the action of heparin in interrupting the coagulation process, "it is logical that prophylaxis against coagulation may be accomplished by small doses of heparin sufficient to inactivate trace quantities of procoagulants high in the coagulation cascade, whereas much larger quantities of heparin are required to interrupt the coagulation scheme once activated factor X and thrombin* are present in high concentrations in the neighborhood of an established clot."

Cardiac Rate and Rhythm.   Sinus tachycardia[15] and sinus bradycardia[7,15,17,35] have both been reported to occur in the early stages of spinal cord injury. Occasional escape rhythms at the onset of injury have also been reported.[17,35] Sinus or junctional bradycardia appear to be mediated by the parasympathetic nervous system.[7,35] In my experience, cervical-spinal cord-injured patients in spinal shock most often exhibit sinus bradycardia that occasionally leads to junctional escape beats or rhythm and rarely, in otherwise healthy individuals, to ventricular beats. These arrhythmias often are more profound when associated with hypothermia or hypoxemia.

There are reports of cardiac arrest in quadraplegic patients initiated by

---

* Heparin inhibits the action of thrombin and activated factor X.

bradycardia produced by a vaso-vagal response to hypoxia.[36–38] Cardiac arrest was subsequently prevented by preoxygenation before suctioning and parasympathetic blockade with atropine. Tracheal suctioning and hypoxia usually produce tachycardia and hypertension in man. Considering the rapidity with which bradycardia and arrest were induced following disconnection from the ventilator, Berk and Levy[36] concluded that the response resembled the primary cardiac reflex response to carotid chemoreceptor stimulation seen in experimental animals. Owing to spinal shock, reflex sympathetic activity below the level of the lesion was not able to produce the usual compensatory responses, and the addition of vagal stimulation by tracheal suctioning led to bradycardia and cardiac arrest (vaso-vagal reflex).[37,38]

Although the number of patients who respond to suctioning in the manner described above are rare, the effects can be fatal, and hyperoxygenation before suctioning and cardiac monitoring are necessary interventions if this complication is to be prevented. Prophylactic use of atropine also has been employed to prevent the vaso-vagal reflex, but caution must be exercised if repeated doses are given.

Poikilothermy.   Spinal cord injury also leads to problems in temperature regulation with cervical-injured patients being in the greatest danger.[6,16,39–41] Spinal cord transection interrupts the sympathetic pathways between the temperature regulating centers in the hypothalamus and the blood vessels. These pathways normally allow for vasodilatation and sweating in hot environments or vasoconstriction and shivering in cold environments. Consequently, spinal cord-injured patients become poikilothermic, i.e., their body temperature rises and falls in response to the environmental temperature.[18]

Serious metabolic strain can occur in hyperthermic environments because the inability to increase heat loss causes these patients to respond by increasing their core temperature, sometimes to alarming levels.[6] Body temperature can be more carefully controlled in air-conditioned units where environmental temperatures can be kept constant. Cheshire[39] reported that hypothermia resulted in this circumstance, but found hypothermia to be desirable because of an approximately 20% decrease in oxygen requirements at a temperature of 34° C. Pledger[40] cited a case of moderately severe hypothermia (30.2° C) with concomitant sinus bradycardia of 40 beats per minute. The patient was confused and uncooperative ''. . . characteristic of hypothermia.'' In my experience, sinus bradycardia and escape rhythms were more prevalent at low body temperatures, and often improved when the patient was warmed toward normal body temperatures. Because cardiac arrhythmias and even ventricular fibrillation may become evident with hypothermia at very low levels,[40,41] the patient's core temperature is usually kept close to normal.

Respiratory Effects

In a review of the causes of acute death (i.e., within 2 months of injury) in spinal cord-injured patients, Tribe[33] reported that respiratory-associated causes were present in 15 of 16 patients. Some of the respiratory effects of acute spinal cord injury have already been discussed (pulmonary embolus and vaso-vagal reflex); others include hypoventilation, pneumonia, and pulmonary edema.

Injury at or above the fourth cervical spinal cord segment will lead to respiratory arrest due to paralysis of all major muscles of respiration, including the diaphragm. Injury below this level may spare the diaphragm and allow the patient some respiratory effort although the vital capacity is decreased, sometimes to as low as 0.1–0.3 liters in the initial stages of spinal shock.[6,18,39,42] Although most quadriplegic patients have a vital capacity and tidal volume adequate to maintain ventilation under basal conditions, they have an ineffective cough, owing to paralysis of abdominal and intercostal muscles, and thus cannot clear the airway of secretions.[39] Stagnation of secretions leads to hypoventilation and respiratory acidosis, and eventually hypoxemia. Hypoxemia leads in turn to intense pulmonary vasoconstriction and edema, which may already be present to some degree as a result of overhydration and cardiovascular insufficiency.[43] The resulting increased work of breathing alters the ventilation-perfusion ratio of the lung. Pulmonary edema or retained secretions can greatly compromise the patient's respiratory ability, since his respiratory reserve is essentially nil as he is using whatever functioning lung tissue he has available. Abdominal distention, which is often present, can further compromise respiratory function by restricting diaphragmatic excursion, thus adding to hypoventilation and hypoxemia.[6] Abdominal distention can also lead to vomiting and pulmonary aspiration and collapse.[39] Any or all complications that lead to hypoventilation or hypoxemia can increase the risk of vaso-vagal reflex response to suctioning.

Atelectasis is caused by gravitational and hydrostatic pressures that tend to encourage collection of secretions in the dependent segments of the lung and may lead to pneumonia.[16,22] Aspiration is also a common complication of high spinal cord injury and leads to a chemical pneumonitis.[42] Endotracheal intubation and tracheostomies offer an easy access route for infection and should be done only when necessary.[16,42]

As previously mentioned, initial assessment of the patient's respiratory status includes a chest x-ray, measurement of tidal volume, vital capacity, and arterial blood gas tensions. These parameters should be monitored closely throughout the early stages of the patient's hospitalization. To prevent retention of secretions in patients who have high thoracic or cervical injuries, frequent turning of the patient, a program of breathing exercises, incentive spirometry, chest percussion, and assisted coughing have proven effective.[44] Adequate humidification, especially when artificial airways are used, is essential in preventing tracheobronchitis.[11,39]

As the flaccid paralysis characteristic of spinal shock converts to the spastic paralysis consistent with upper motor neuron lesions, the pulmonary function of the patient should improve. This improvement is related to more effective diaphragmatic contraction aided by the increased muscle tone of the abdominal and intercostal muscles.[44] If atelectasis and pneumonia have been successfully prevented with the above regimen, it is possible, in many cases, to avoid intubation or tracheotomizing of the patient.[44]

Pulmonary Edema. Pulmonary edema has been reported as a complication and cause of death in cervical spinal cord injury. Fluid overload is implicated as the cause in many cases, since patients are frequently resuscitated with large volumes of fluid in an effort to treat hypotension. Overtransfusion often occurs in the spinal cord-injured patient because rapid infusion raises the blood pressure only slightly in the face of sympathetic paralysis.[16] Fluid overload occurred most frequently in patients who were initially resuscitated by medical and nursing personnel unaccustomed to caring for acute spinal injuries,[39] or in patients with multiple injuries and hemorrhage.[15,16] Silver[43] pointed out that pulmonary edema can also result from a tendency for fluid to collect in the lungs as a manifestation of generalized fluid retention in the early stages of injury. Patients with high cervical injuries have a decreased vital capacity which, if severe enough to cause hypoxemia, may result in pulmonary vasoconstriction with respiratory failure and edema.[43]

There have been case reports of apparent neurogenic pulmonary edema. The most striking case was that of a 15-year-old boy who sustained a spinal cord transection at the fifth cervical segment and developed pulmonary edema 11 hours after injury. There were no other mechanisms, such as head trauma, fluid overload, chest trauma, or cardiac disease, that could explain the development of pulmonary edema.[45] Animal experiments suggest that central nervous system lesions causing an increase in intracranial pressure produce sympathetic discharge, which in turn causes increased total peripheral resistance, decreased cardiac output, and increased left atrial pressure—all resulting in acute pulmonary congestion. Poe, Reisman, and Rodenhouse[45] suggest that "upper spinal cord injury may cause a sudden increase in intracranial pressure and a massive sympathetic outpouring or a hormonal response." Experimental studies have supported this hypothesis. Brisman et al.[46] demonstrated a rise in pulmonary artery wedge pressure in dogs with spinal cord transection when infused with fluid and catecholamines. In experimental animals, compression of the spinal cord by ligature to obstruct cerebrospinal fluid flow led to increased blood pressure due to increased cardiac output, bradycardia, and increased pulmonary artery and pulmonary wedge pressures, which in turn were possibly due to sympathetic stimulation.[47] Other authors agree that while there may indeed be a neurogenic pulmonary edema produced by cervical spinal cord injury, the picture has often been clouded by factors such as chest injury or increased blood and plasma volumes from overtransfusion.[15,22,32] Pulmonary edema associated with spinal cord injury is rare, and the mechanism remains unclear.[48]

Because of the serious nature of this complication, efforts aimed at prevention, early detection, and treatment are imperative. Again, it must be emphasized that this patient's respiratory reserve is minimal and that the normal clinical response to fluid replacement is absent, owing to lack of sympathetic tone. Fluid replacement should be guided by hemodynamic monitoring. Chest auscultation will detect the presence of rales, an early sign of pulmonary edema. Frequent assessment of arterial blood gases, calculation of alveolar-arterial oxygen difference, and measurement of the patient's pulmonary compliance will aid in determining his oxygenation status.

Gastrointestinal Effects

Gastric Dilatation and Ileus. Gastric dilatation and ileus are common signs exhibited by spinal cord-injured patients[6,39,43] and are due to loss of central control.[6] As pointed out earlier, gastric dilatation can interfere with diaphragmatic function causing hypoventilation, and may lead to hypoxemia. In addition, vomiting with resultant pulmonary aspiration can occur, and occasionally leads to sudden death from respiratory failure.[6] Vomiting and aspiration may be prevented by the insertion of a nasogastric tube attached to low intermittent suction.[49] However, the removal of gastric contents can lead to metabolic alkalosis from loss of chloride and hydrogen ions,[39] as well as to potassium deficit, therefore appropriate replacement should be given intravenously. Extracellular volume deficit can also occur with prolonged gastrointestinal suction and further complicate the existing hypotension. Cheshire[39] pointed out that potassium losses after spinal cord injury may be high; failure to restore potassium deficits leads both to impairment of cardiac and smooth muscle function and to extracellular hyponatremia and intracellular sodium loading.

Stress Ulcers. Numerous reports can be found in the literature of stress ulcers occurring in seriously ill or injured patients. Many authors categorize these ulcers according to cause, which suggests a different physiologic pathway for each.[50–54] All agree that Cushing's ulcer, one type of stress ulcer, is associated with serious brain lesions and seems to be characterized by high gastric acid output, possibly mediated by vagal stimulation. A Cushing's ulcer may involve the esophagus, stomach, and duodenum. Cervical-spinal cord-injured patients are probably candidates for Cushing's ulcer. Guttman[5] stated that ". . . interruption of the vasoconstrictors in the spinal cord results in paralytic vasodilatation, leading to mucosal hemorrhage forming necrotic areas, eventually causing ulceration." He as well as others,[11,49,55] agree that stress ulceration may be the result of vagal-stimulated gastric acid production and/or release of adrenocorticotropic hormone (ACTH).

Steroids are often used as part of the treatment regimen in acute spinal cord injury, and have been implicated in the production of stress ulcers.[16,54,56] However, there is evidence to suggest that short-term pharmacologic doses of steroids actually decrease the incidence of gastric ulceration in patients with hemorrhagic shock. Jama, Perlman, and Matsumoto[53] found a 5.9% incidence of gastric ulcers in shock patients who were given pharmacologic doses of steroids, and a 57.9% incidence in patients treated for hemorrhagic shock without steroids. Whether this information can be applied to patients with spinal cord injury is not known. Epstein, Hood, and Ransohoff[57] reported 20.9% incidence of gastrointestinal bleeding in patients receiving high doses of steroids (methylprednisolone 1 gm per day) and 16.7% incidence in those receiving low doses of steroids (methylprednisolone 160 mg per day).

The incidence of stress ulcers associated with spinal cord injury is difficult to determine. Meinecke[16] reported that he had not seen stress ulcers in his spinal cord-injured patients, but others report a 20–22% incidence of gastrointestinal bleeding in patients with spinal cord lesions.[55,57] Moody and Cheung[51] found that fiberoptic gastroscopy revealed a higher-than-expected incidence of ulceration in burn patients although the incidence of bleeding was low.

Gastric ulcers present a significant threat to the spinal cord-injured patients because of the potential for hemorrhage, which is frequently the initial manifestation of stress ulcer.[50,51,56] Hemorrhage is sometimes severe enough to cause shock, which these patients are ill prepared to combat (lacking the usual sympathetic compensatory mechanism), and mortality reports vary between 15 and 50%.[51,56]

Cimetidine and antacids have been advocated in the prevention and treatment of ulcers.[58,59] Cimetidine inhibits gastric acid secretion by acting as a specific competitive histamine H_2-receptor antagonist.[60] Histamine increases gastric acid secretion and acidity; the acid is able to penetrate the (mucosal) barrier and leads to development of ischemic cells.[52] Burland and Parr[58] concluded from their study of 119 patients with gastric hemorrhage that "cimetidine has a place in the management of patients bleeding from ulceration or erosions of the esophagus, stomach, or duodenum." Prophylactic administration of antacids to maintain a neutral luminal pH is a common and effective method for the prevention of gastric ulcerations.[51,59] In a study of 131 spinal cord-injured patients, Epstein, Hood, and Ransohoff[57] found that cimetidine plus antacids did not offer significantly better prevention or control of GI bleeding than antacids alone.

In addition to cimetidine and antacids, the treatment of gastric bleeding includes gastric lavage. Both cold and warm saline have been used, and in about 80% of cases, this alone will stop the bleeding.[51] Coagulation defects should be checked for and a unit of fresh whole blood should be given every sixth unit of blood transfusion to provide adequate clotting factors. Intraarterial infusion of vasopressin via the left gastric artery has been successfully used with uncontrollable bleeding.[51] Occasional surgery (vagotomy and pyloroplasty or gastrectomy) may be necessary.[51] Again, it must be pointed out that the spinal cord-injured patient is a poor surgical risk, especially in the first few weeks after injury.

Urinary System

A problem that can have serious consequences in the spinal cord injured patient is atony of the bladder. The bladder does not contract and the paralyzed detrusor muscle does not open, resulting in urinary retention.[5,47,61] Urinary retention can cause urinary infection, reflux, stone formation and upper urinary tract back pressure leading to renal deterioration.[61] Treatment by intermittent catherization is highly recommended in an effort to decrease the incidence of urinary tract infections associated with indwelling catheters.[6,16,49,61] An indwelling catheter may be necessary in the first few days after injury, however, if the patient is hypotensive and requires careful monitoring of his fluid status. Urinary tract infections can occasionally lead to septic shock and oliguria with renal deterioration[61]; therefore, attempts at prevention of infection, early detection, and treatment with appropriate antibiotic therapy are mandatory. Infections can greatly prolong the state of spinal shock and ultimately the patient's recovery and function.[6]

Psychological Effects

The complexity of the reactions of patients and families to the disaster of sudden spinal cord transection is beyond the scope of this discussion. A multitude of references on the subject are available for a more complete discussion regarding the stages these patients must move through toward recovery of psychological health. A few brief suggestions are made here to assist in the initial care of the patient.

Guttmann[6] stated, "The sudden conversion of a vigorous person into a helpless wreck, naturally leads to severe psychological shock." He pointed out that initially the patient is incapable of realizing the extent of his or her disability, and perception may be impaired by drugs, tramatic shock, hypoxemia, and associated injuries. Meinecke[16] emphasized the importance of honesty in dealing with the patient and his family regarding the patient's altered state and prognosis, and pointed to the value of a positive attitude by the nurses and physicians. Active participation of the patient in his own care is very important and can be accomplished in the initial stages of injury by allowing the patient to make decisions, however small, regarding his care. Defining and setting appropriate limits of behavior will do much in alleviating the dependent, demanding behavior these patients are inclined to develop. Pepper[62] advocated consistency in meeting the physical needs of the patient, which aids in establishing the patient's sense of trust and sets limits that provide predictability.

Treatment

Many factors have been implicated as causative or contributory in the histopathologic changes that occur from spinal cord injury. There is evidence that decreased spinal cord blood flow occurs within hours of injury and may be responsible for ischemic changes.[63–65] These changes may be mediated by a loss of autoregulation, progressive edema causing small vessel compression, decreased tissue oxygen levels, and/or release of vasoactive substances such as norepinephrine, dopamine, or serotonin.[63–65] Trauma and resulting ischemia and edema may have damaging effects on cell membranes, as evidenced by decreased Na^+-K^+-activated ATPase, and may reflect altered platelet function.[66] Potassium depletion and increased sodium concentration in the injured cord have been documented, along with progressive edema.[67]

As a result of these and other studies, therapeutic efforts mostly involving experimental animals have been directed at preventing or reversing these effects. There appears to be agreement that adequate immobilization immediately after injury and institution of therapy within 4 hours of injury are necessary if treatment is to be effective.[7,68] Ducker, Saleman, and Daniel[69] reported that immobilization alone was as effective in recovery of function as administration of any one of five pharmacologic agents (dextran, phenobarbital, methyldopa, phenoxybenzamine, and vasopressors) advocated in recent years for treating spinal cord injuries. Early surgery for stabilization of the spine is more controversial, but there seems to be a consensus that it is indicated for removal of bony fragments or intraspinal discs.[7]

Hypothermia of the injured cord has been studied extensively and there are many conflicting reports. Wells and Hansebout[70] found that 4 hours of cooling of the spinal cord without opening the dura resulted in greater function in dogs. Tator and Deecke[71] reported that perfusion of the spinal cord with normothermic normal saline was of more benefit in recovery of monkeys than durotomy or hypothermic perfusion, perhaps because of dialysis of noxious substances. In 1973, Meacham and McPherson treated 14 clinically complete spinal cord-injured patients with local hypothermia and reported return of function in 7 and ambulation in 3 patients. They have since discontinued treating patients in this manner, however, because they have found no significant difference in recovery in comparison to patients not so treated.[13] Thienprasit et al.[71] found that cats treated with both laminectomy and delayed hypothermia (6 hours post-injury) improved more than those treated only with laminectomy. They also found that if somatosensory evoked potentials returned within 6 hours of injury, the animals recovered, whether or not they were treated.

Glucocorticoids have been used alone and with other forms of therapy in spinal cord injury. The mechanism by which glucocorticoids are thought to exert their therapeutic effects probably involve stabilization of the capillary endothelial membrane, maintenance of intracellular potassium, and preservation of lysosomal and membrane bound enzymes.[11] In animals given "threshold" (amount of trauma necessary to produce paralysis) spinal cord lesions, the greatest recovery over a 7-week period was in dogs treated with both steroids (dexamethasone) and local hypothermia.[73] Because the lesions were produced by compression rather than impact, the results are difficult to correlate to traumatic spinal cord injury in humans. Ducker and Hamit[12] found that intramuscular dexamethasone or local hypothermia was more effective in recovery of injury dogs than was intrathecal methylprednisolone. Lewin, Hansebout, and Pappius[67] demonstrated a significantly better functional recovery in cats treated with dexamethasone than in control animals and attributed this finding to prevention of loss of potassium from the injured cord. Bucy[10] advocated immediate immobilization and steroid administration in spinal cord-injured patients. Green, Kahn, and Klose[11] studied the effects of methylprednisolone and dexamethasone on experimentally produced spinal cord injury in monkeys. They found no difference in outcome between the two steroids, but reported that there was statistically significant differences in the clinical improvement between treated and untreated animals, although not to the point of a cure. They concluded that glucocorticoid administration "might play a beneficial role" in the treatment of spinal cord injury. Albin[7] reported, however, that no substantial data have emerged to indicate the efficacy of steroids in the treatment of humans with spinal cord injuries.

In attempting to prevent ischemic changes from taking place, Hedeman and Sil[23] studied the effects of various pharmacologic agents. They found that phenoxybenzamine, an alpha-adrenergic blocking agent, offered protection from paralysis in dogs. Haloperidol and low-molecular-weight dextran, thought to prevent rises in dopamine levels, had a lesser effect, and steroids and alpha-methyltyrosine were not effective at all. Senter, Venes, and Kauer[75] found that gamma-hydroxybutyrate, a central nervous system (CNS) depressant that may interfere with the release or activation of several vasoactive substances, markedly altered the ischemic response to injury in cats if given in the early post-traumatic period. Recall that Ducker et al.[69] found no beneficial effect from dextran, phenobarbital, methyldopa, phenoxybenzamine, or vasopressors when compared with immobilization in experimental spinal cord injury.

SUMMARY

The problems of acute spinal cord-injured patients are many. The cardiovascular, respiratory, gastrointestinal, and urinary problems frequently encountered have been described with reference to the acid-base and fluid and electrolyte disorders that result. Reference was made to the psychological aspects, and current concepts in treatment were discussed. Nursing care of these patients is of primary importance, as was pointed out by Bucy and Perot,[76] "Without intelligent, adequately educated, and trained nurses, all else will fail. They are absolutely essential to the success in this difficult area."

REFERENCES

1. Mesard L: Survival after spinal cord trauma. Arch Neurol 35:78–83, 1978.
2. Guttmann L: Spinal cord injuries: Comprehensive management and research. Blackwell Scientific Publications, Oxford, 1976.
3. McCough, G: Physiology of the spinal cord. In Austin G, Ed: The spinal cord. Charles C. Thomas, Springfield, 1972.
4. Larrebee JH: The person with a spinal cord injury. Physical care during early recovery. Am J Nurs 77: 1320, 1977.
5. Osterholm JL: The pathophysiological response to spinal cord injury. J Neurosurg 40:5–33, 1974.
6. Guttmann L: Spinal shock. In Vinken PJ and Bruyn GW, Eds: Handbook of Clinical Neurology. Injuries of the spine and spinal cord. Part II. pp. 243–262. American Elsevier, New York, 1976.
7. Albin MS: Resuscitation of the spinal cord. Crit Care Med 6:270–276, 1978.
8. Roberts JR: Trauma of the cervical spine. Top Em Med 1:63–77, 1979.
9. Yeo JD: First aid management of spinal cord injuries. Med J Aust 2:531–532, 1979.
10. Bucy PC: Emergency treatment of spinal cord injury (editorial). Surg Neurol 1:216, 1973.
11. Green B, Kahn T, and Klose KJ: A comparative study of steroid therapy in acute experimental spinal cord injury. Surg Neurol 13:91–97, 1980.
12. Ducker TB and Hamit HF: Experimental treatments of acute spinal cord injury. J Neurosurg 30:693–697, 1969.

13. Botterell EH: Acute cord injury. Parts I & II. J R Coll Surg Edin 23:57–64, 107–117, 1978.
14. Guttmann L: Total responsibility of the surgeon in the management of traumatic spinal paraplegics and tetraplegics. Paraplegia 15:285–292, 1977–78.
15. Meyer GA, et al: Hemodynamic responses to acute quadriplegia with or without chest trauma. J Neurosurg 34:168, 1971.
16. Meinecke FW: Initial clinical appraisal. In Vinken PJ and Bruyn GW, Eds: Handbook of Clinical Neurology. Injuries of the spine and spinal cord. Part II. pp. 202–242. American Elsevier, New York, 1976.
17. Tibbs PA, et al: Studies of experimental cervical cord transection. Part I: Hemodynamic changes after acute cervical cord transection. J Neurosurg 49:558, 1978.
18. Tsai SH, Shih CJ, Shyy TT, and Liu JC: Recovery of vasomotor response in human spinal cord transection. J Neurosurg 52:808–811, 1980.
19. Braunwald E: Regulation of the circulation. Part II. N Engl J Med 290:1420–1425, 1974.
20. McKibbin B and Brotherton BJ: The early management of cervical spine injuries. Resuscitation 2:241, 1973.
21. Silver JR: Vascular reflexes in spinal shock. Paraplegia 8:231, 1971.
22. Bellamy R, Pitts FW, Stauffer ES: Respiratory complications in traumatic quadraplegia. J Neurosurg 39:596, 1973.
23. Rawe SE, Lee WA, and Perot PL: The histopathology of experimental spinal cord trauma. The effect of systemic blood pressure. J Neurosurg 48:1002–1007, 1978.
24. Alderman JL, Osterholm JL, D'Amore BR, et al: Influence of arterial blood pressure upon central hemorrhagic necrosis after severe spinal cord injury. Neurosurg 4:53–55, 1979.
25. Frankel HL, and Mathias CJ: The cardiovascular system in tetraplegia and paraplegia. In Vinken PJ and Bruyn GW Eds: Handbook of Clinical Neurology. Injuries of the spine and spinal cord. Part II. pp. 313–328. American Elsevier, New York, 1976.
26. Casas ER, et al: Prophylaxis of venous thrombosis and pulmonary embolism in patients with acute traumatic spinal cord lesions. Paraplegia 15:209–214, 1977.
27. Silver JR and Moulton A: The physiological and pathological sequelae of paralysis of intercostal and abdominal muscles in tetraplegic patients. Paraplegia 7:131, 1969.
28. Watson N: Anticoagulant therapy in the treatment of venous thrombosis and pulmonary embolism in acute spinal injury. Paraplegia 12:197–201, 1974.
29. Watson N: Anti-coagulant therapy in the prevention of venous thrombosis and pulmonary emboli in the spinal cord injury. Paraplegia 16:265–269, 1978–79.
30. Perkash A, Prakash V, and Perkash I: Experience with the management of thromboembolism in patients with spinal cord injury: Part I. Incidence, diagnosis, and role of some risk factors. Paraplegia 16:322–331, 1978–79.
31. Silver JR: The prophylactic use of anticoagulant therapy in the prevention of pulmonary emboli in one hundred consecutive spinal injury patients. Paraplegia 12:188–196, 1974.
32. Tribe CR: Causes of death in the early stage of paraplegia. Paraplegia 1:19, 1963.
33. Nicolaides AN and Hobbs JT: Diagnosis of venous thrombosis by the ^{125}I-fibrinogen test. In Bergan J and Yao J, Eds: Venous Problems. Yearbook Medical Publishers, Chicago, 1978.
34. Salzman EW: Heparin therapy in venous thromboembolism. In Bergan J and Yao J, Eds: Venous Problems, Yearbook Medical Publishers, Chicago, 1978.

35. Evans DE, Kobrine AI, Rizzoli HV: Cardiac arrhythmias accompanying acute compression of the spinal cord. J Neurosurg 52:52–59, 1980.
36. Berk JL and Levy MN: Profound reflex bradycardia produced by transient hypoxia or hypercapnia in man. Eur Surg Res 9:75, 1977.
37. Frankel HL, Mathias CJ, and Spaulding JMK: Mechanisms of reflex cardiac arrest in tetraplegic patients. Lancet ii:1183, 1975 (Dec. 13).
38. Dollfus P and Frankel HL: Cardiovascular reflexes in tracheostomized tetraplegics. Paraplegia 2:227, 1965.
39. Cheshire DJE: Respiratory and metabolic management in acute tetraplegia. Paraplegia 4:1, 1966.
40. Pledger HG: Disorders of temperature regulation in acute traumatic tetraplegia. J Bone Joint Surg 44B:110, 1962.
41. Johnson RH: Temperature regulation. In Vinken PJ and Bruyn GW, Eds: Handbook of Clinical Neurology. Injuries of the spine and spinal cord. Part II. pp. 355–372. American Elsevier, New York, 1976.
42. Fugl-Meyer AR: The respiratory system. In Vinken PJ and Bruyn GW, Eds: Handbook of Clinical Neurology. Injuries of the spine and spinal cord. Part II. pp. 335–347. American Elsevier, New York, 1976.
43. Silver JR: Chest injuries and complications in the early stages of spinal cord injury. Paraplegia 5:226, 1968.
44. McMichan JC, Michel L, Westbrook PR: Pulmonary dysfunction following traumatic quadriplegia. JAMA 243:528–531, 1980.
45. Poe RH, Reisman JL, and Rodenhouse TG: Pulmonary edema in cervical spinal cord injury. J Trauma 18:71–73, 1978.
46. Brisman R, et al: Pulmonary edema in acute transection of the cervical spinal cord. Surg Gynecol Obstet 139:363–366, 1974.
47. Miner ME, Gonzales NC, and Overman J: Cardiovascular response to independent cephalic and spinal cord pressure elevations. Surg Forum 23:407–409, 1972.
48. Graf CJ and Rossi NP: Pulmonary edema and the central nervous system: A clinicopathological study. Surg Neurol 4:319–324, 1978.
49. Burke DC and Murray DD: Handbook of spinal cord medicine. pp. 26–46. Raven Press, New York, 1975.
50. Price SA and Wilson LM: Stomach and duodenum. In Pathophysiology: Clinical Concepts of Disease Process. pp. 206–219. McGraw Hill, New York, 1978.
51. Moody FG and Cheung LY: Stress ulcers: Their pathogenesis, diagnosis, and prevention. Surg Clin North Am 56:1469–1478, 1976.
52. Kawarada Y, Lambek J, and Matsumoto T: Pathophysiology of stress ulcer and its prevention. Am J Surg 129:217–222, 1975.
53. Jama RH, Perlman MH, and Matsumoto T: Incidence of stress ulcer formation associated with steroid therapy in various shock states. Am J Surg 130:328–331, 1975.
54. Markowitz AM: Acute gastrointestinal problems in the intensive care unit. Med Clin North Am 55:1277, 1971.
55. Perret G and Solomon A: Gastrointestinal hemorrhage and cervical cord injuries. Proceedings 17th VA Spinal Cord Injury Conferences , pp. 106–110. New York, 1969.
56. Nuseibeh IM: Stress ulceration in spinal injuries. In Vinken PJ and Bruyn GW, Eds: Handbook of Clinical Neurology. Injuries of the spine and spinal cord. Part II, pp. 351–353. American Elsivier, New York, 1976.

57. Epstein N, Hood DC, Ransohoff J: Gastrointestinal bleeding in patients with spinal cord trauma. J Neurosurg 54:16–20, 1981.
58. Burland WL and Parr SN: Experiences with cemetidine in the treatment of seriously ill patients. In Burland WL and Simkins F, Eds: International Symposium on Histamine H_2-Receptor Antagonists. Excerpta Medica, Amsterdam, 1977.
59. Strauss RJ, et al: Cemetidine, carbenoxolone sodium, and antacids for the prevention of experimental stress ulcers. Arch Surg 113:858–862, 1978.
60. Brogden RN, et al: Cemetidine: A review of its pharmacological properties and therapeutic efficiency in peptic ulcer disease. Drugs 15: 93–131, 1978.
61. O'Flynn JD: Early management of neuropathic bladder in spinal cord injuries. Paraplegia 12:83, 1974.
62. Pepper GA: A person with a spinal cord injury: Psychological care. Am J Nurs 77:1330–1336, 1977.
63. Senter HJ and Venes JL: Altered blood flow and secondary injury in experimental spinal cord trauma. J Neurosurg 49:569–578, 1978.
64. Senter HJ and Venes JL: Loss of autoregulation and posttraumatic ischemia following experimental spinal cord trauma. J Neurosurg 50:198–206, 1979.
65. Ducker TB, et al: Experimental spinal cord trauma. I. Correlation of blood flow, tissue oxygen and neurologic status in the dog. Surg Neurol 10:60–63, 1978.
66. Clendenon NR: Inhibition of Na^+-K^+-activated ATPase activity following experimental spinal cord trauma. J Neurosurg 49:563–568, 1978.
67. Lewin MG, Hansebout RR, and Pappius HM: Chemical characteristics of traumatic spinal cord edema in cats. Effects of steroids on potassium depletion. J Neurosurg 40:65, 1974.
68. Bucy, PC: Immediate immobilization of fractured spines (editorial). Surg Neurol 10:63, 1978.
69. Ducker TB, Saleman M, and Daniell HB: Experimental spinal cord trauma. III. Therapeutic effects of immobilization and pharmacologic agents. Surg Neurol 10:71–76, 1978.
70. Wells JD, and Hansebout RR: Local hypothermia in experimental spinal cord trauma. Surg Neurol 10:200–204, 1978.
71. Tator CH and Deecke L: Value of normothermic perfusion, hypothermic perfusion, and durotomy in the treatment of experimental acute spinal cord trauma. J Neurosurg 39:52–63, 1973.
72. Thienprasit P: Effect of delayed local cooling on experimental spinal cord injury. J Neurosurg 42:150–154, 1975.
73. Kuchner EF and Hansebout RR: Combined steroid and hypothermia treatment of experimental spinal cord injury. Surg Neurol 6:371–376, 1976.
74. Hedeman LS, and Sil R: Studies in experimental spinal cord trauma. Part 2. Comparison of treatment with steroids, low molecular weight dextran, and catecholamine blockade. J Neurosurg 40:44–50, 1974.
75. Senter HJ, Venes JL, and Kauer JS: Alteration of posttraumatic ischemia in experimental spinal cord trauma by a central nervous system depressant. J Neurosurg 50:207–216, 1979.
76. Bucy PC and Perot PL: Injury to the spinal cord. In Tower DB, Ed: The Nervous System. Vol. 2. The Clinical Neurosciences. Raven Press, New York, 1975.

7 | Status Epilepticus

Mary Pat Lovely
Judy Ozuna

Status epilepticus (SE) is a medical emergency that may be encountered in any critical care area. It is a serious condition which can lead to metabolic and physical exhaustion and even death. Thus, SE requires intensive care and observation to prevent devastating sequelae. The needs of the patient can best be met by understanding the mechanism, treatment methods, and complications of repeated seizures.

DEFINITIONS

Status epilepticus has been defined in many different ways. Browne defined it as seizures persisting for 30 minutes or longer.[1] Celesia defined it as a seizure persisting for at least 30 minutes or, as defined by the International League Against Epilepsy, "is repeated frequently enough to produce a fixed and enduring epileptic condition" lasting at least 30 minutes.[2] This is often interpreted to include persons who do not regain consciousness between successive seizures.

There are several types of seizures, any of which can be manifested in SE. The International Classification of Seizures[3] divides them into generalized and partial, based on clinical and electroencephalographic manifestations. Generalized seizures involve the whole brain and include tonic-clonic (grand mal), solely tonic, solely clonic, typical absence (petit mal), atypical absence, myoclonic, and akinetic seizures. Partial seizures involve only a part of the brain and include those seizures with elementary symptomatology (focal motor or focal sensory phenomena) and those with complex symptomatology (psychomotor or temporal lobe phenomena). The most common and most life-threatening form of SE is generalized tonic-clonic (grand mal).

CAUSES OF STATUS EPILEPTICUS

In several patient series, over half the cases of SE in adults were symptomatic of other diseases.[2,4,5] Among these diseases were cerebral tumors (especially in the frontal regions), cerebrovascular disease, infection (meningitis, encephalitis), head trauma, metabolic disorders, and drug abuse (alcohol, barbiturates).[2,4,6] In patients with epilepsy, the most common cause of SE was failure to take anticonvulsant drugs regularly.[5-7]

In children, the causes of SE are somewhat different. Cryptogenic causes accounted for 126 of the 239 cases in children under 15 years of age described by Aicardi and Chevrie.[8] Sixty-seven of the 126 cases were associated with fever. Acute brain injury (meningitis, encephalitis, subdural hematoma, dehydration and electrolyte disorders, anoxic injury, and exogenous toxins) and chronic encephalopathy (birth injury, progressive and nonprogressive encephalopathy, congenital brain defects) were the most common symptomatic causes of SE in this patient series.

SIGNIFICANCE

The mortality rate of SE rises as the duration of seizures increases and may rise as high as 20%.[4,5] Death may be due to the complications of SE or to the underlying pathology, e.g., brain tumor. Patients in the latter group often respond poorly to conventional treatment and account for all the deaths that occurred during the acute phase of SE in one series.[4] Rowan[5] noted definite anoxic brain damage, probably due to SE itself, on postmortem examination in three patients who had SE. Morbidity has been reported as 12.5–26% in adults[5,6] and 37% in children.[8] Morbidity in SE is highest in infants and decreases with age. The incidence of tonic-clonic SE in patients with a history of epilepsy is 1–5% and accounts for one third of all epilepsy-related deaths.[1]

Because a poorer prognosis is associated with increased duration of SE[4,6] and may lead to death, it is imperative to initiate vigorous measures to stop the seizure, to maintain vital functions, and to prevent traumatic injury.[1]

INITIAL TREATMENT

Several actions are initiated in all cases of SE. Respiratory and ECG monitoring are required. An intravenous line is inserted for administration of fluid and drugs. Blood should be analyzed for glucose, sodium, potassium, calcium, phosphorous, magnesium, and blood urea nitrogen, as well as for anticonvulsant drug levels and toxic substances (e.g., alcohol, lead). Blood cultures should be done if sepsis is suspected. Remember that hyperpyrexia accompanies tonic-clonic SE and is not always a sign of septicemia. A complete blood count should also be done as anemia is seen with lead poisoning, sickle cell disease, and leukemia, each of which may be associated with seizures.

Leukocytosis is often found in response to the stress of the seizure and does not necessarily imply the presence of an underlying infection.[9]

If SE does not respond readily to treatment, a urinary catheter and a nasogastric tube should be inserted. Intake and output should be monitored and urine should be cultured and examined for myoglobin and toxic substances. The stomach may be emptied via the nasogastric tube, thus preventing aspiration of vomitus or secretions, which leads to a chemical pneumonitis and immediate respiratory compromise.

The seizure manifestations themselves must be carefully observed, for they can give valuable clues to the diagnosis of the type and cause of SE. Signs that the seizure is lateralized to one side should be noted. If the head and eyes deviate, they usually move toward the side opposite the seizure focus until the muscles tire, when they then move either medially or toward the seizure focus.[10] The nature and quality of motor movements should be observed. Any asymmetry in the movements of the limbs should be noted, as they may imply a focal lesion. General neurologic function should be assessed and monitored throughout the episode of SE; this includes level of consciousness (particularly between attacks), pupil size, equality, and reactivity, and gross motor and sensory function.

The person in SE must also be examined for evidence of head trauma, bruises and/or fractures of the body and limbs, and for needle marks. The latter may indicate drug abuse and may indicate the cause of SE.

SYSTEMIC RESPONSES IN SE AND TREATMENT OF ASSOCIATED COMPLICATIONS

Cerebral

During a seizure, many action potentials in single cells occur in rapid succession (high frequency bursts).[11] This intense neuronal activity places a heavy metabolic demand on the cells, and high energy phosphate compounds (upon which cells depend for energy) decline rapidly leading to failure of the Na-K-ATPase pump.[12] A two to threefold increase in cerebral metabolic rate,[13] oxygen and glucose utilization, and glycolysis[14] occurs. Cellular respiration must increase in order to resynthesize the high energy phosphate compounds and neurotransmitter substances which are consumed during this increased neuronal activity.[10]

Because of the increased energy demands, cerebral blood flow increases three to five times in order to supply oxygen and glucose to the brain.[12] This increase in blood flow results from the increase in arterial pressure and massive dilatation of cerebral resistance vessels, which results from the effects of accumulated CO_2 and lactic acid. These cerebral vascular changes may or may not be compensatory. In baboons with chemically induced SE,[13] increased cerebral blood flow compensated for both a drop in arterial oxygenation and an increase in metabolic demand in the initial phase of SE. However, autoregulation of cerebral blood flow ceases to be effective as SE continues, and cerebral vessels dilate and arterial pressure falls leading to inadequate cerebral perfusion.[12]

In the presence of adequate oxygenation, the brain is able to increase the rate of oxidative metabolism to compensate for the increased energy requirements.[12] In a study of induced SE in rats that were oxygenated and kept normotensive and normoglycemic, a new "steady state" of cerebral metabolism was reached. In another study of mice with induced SE and controlled ventilation, the usual decline in high energy phosphate compounds also was absent.[15] On the other hand, when the oxygen supply was insufficient the rate of glycolysis increased in an attempt to compensate, but lactate accumulated instead of being further metabolized and, along with increased CO_2, led to acidosis.[12]

A serious consequence of SE is sequelae from neuronal damage.[12,16–18] In a study of induced SE in baboons, the areas of brain most affected were small pyramidal cells in the neocortex and hippocampus of the cerebrum and Purkinje's cells in the cerebellum.[19] This brain damage became evident during the second phase of the SE when hyperpyrexia, mild arterial hypotension, mild systemic hypoxia, and acidosis were characteristically seen, and severe hypoglycemia was occasionally seen. Meldrum[18] later provided strong evidence that cerebellar damage was the result of arterial hypotension and hyperpyrexia, while damage to the neocortex and hippocampus was due to the intensity and duration of the seizure discharge itself. He demonstrated that astrocytes became swollen during excessive neuronal activity, owing to the osmotic effects from uptake of increased amounts of metabolic byproducts (lactate, amino acids, ammonia) and postulated that this swelling could be impaired transport of substrates and metabolites to and from active neurons, thus causing ischemic cell damage.

Children in SE are more susceptible to brain damage than adults. In adults, brain damage is usually produced only when seizures exceed 6 hours in duration, but in infants and small children brain damage can follow seizures lasting only 1–2 hours.[19] The special vulnerability of the immature brain to SE has been substantiated by experimental studies in young rats[20] and by clinical studies in children.[8] Duffy[21] suggested that the metabolic demands of the seizures reduce the brain/blood glucose ratio, which may irrevocably disrupt protein metabolism and growth. The permanence of this damage necessitates vigorous attempts to control seizures and the accompanying physiological changes (hypoxia, hyperpyrexia, hypotension, hypoglycemia).

Respiratory

There are a variety of mechanisms by which seizure activity leads to ventilatory insufficiency and hypoxemia.[12] Seizures have a depressant effect on brainstem respiratory centers, and apnea may occur during the tonic phase of seizure activity. In addition, increased total body oxygen consumption may increase beyond respiratory capabilities. Meldrum[13] found that respiratory acidosis occurred within the first 30 minutes of chemically induced SE in baboons. A third mechanism that alters respiratory function is peripheral parasympathetic discharge which creates bronchial constriction and increased secretions. In some species sympathetic discharge can produce hemorrhagic consolidation of the lungs.[13]

Respiratory function can also be compromised by aspiration of vomitus or secretions. Positioning in the semiprone position may improve the airway. If the jaw is sufficiently relaxed, an oral airway should be inserted. Oxygen can be delivered via nasal prongs at 3 liters per minute. While there are no set rules regarding intubation and assisted ventilation, the decision is guided by the patency of the airway, the quality and quantity of respirations, presence of pallor or cyanosis, and blood gas values. One clinician reported that it was seldom necessary to resort to intubation,[23] whereas others preferred to intubate and artificially ventilate patients in tonic-clonic SE immediately. Overmedication with anticonvulsant drugs may impair respiration ability enough to require assisted ventilation.

Cardiovascular

During the initial phase of SE (the first 20–30 minutes), arterial blood pressure rises. This may be due to excessive motor activity and increased venous return, but is probably the result of stimulation of chemoreceptors in the aortic arch and carotid bodies by hypoxia or hypercarbia, causing stimulation of the vasomotor center leading to vasoconstriction. After 30 minutes of SE, there is commonly a drop in the mean arterial pressure to below normal that may persist in the postictal phase.[19] This is apparently due to a drop in peripheral vascular resistance and cardiac output.

Hyperkalemia may develop due to excessive muscular activity or from phenytoin toxicity and may result in cardiac arrhythmias. Bradycardia and/or tachycardia also may be the result of excessive autonomic discharge during SE.

An increase in hematocrit (hemoconcentration) may occur early in generalized tonic-clonic seizures, due to autonomically mediated increased fluid secretion (saliva, tracheo-bronchial secretions, gastric secretions) and perhaps in part to release of splenic reserves of red blood cells.[19]

Restoration of cardiovascular function can be achieved by adequate oxygenation and simultaneous correction of acidosis, hypovolemia, and electrolyte imbalances. This should be done *before* the administration of anticonvulsant drugs, as these drugs are more toxic under conditions of hypoxia and acidosis.[24] Isotonic solutions such as lactated Ringer's or normal saline solutions are preferred for resuscitation to avoid producing cerebral edema. Solutions containing glucose are often given to provide a small but consistant amount of glucose to meet the metabolic needs of the brain.

Metabolic

In Meldrum's baboon study,[13] metabolic acidosis due to increased lactate concentration from excessive muscular activity occurred within the first 30 minutes of induced SE. This was accompanied by hyperglycemia, probably owing to glycolysis and gluconeogenesis. Hyperpyrexia and hyperkalemia, owing to muscular activity, occurred after 30 minutes of SE and was accompanied by normal lactate concentration and normal or low glucose. Once low, the glucose level did not spontaneously recover. Meldrum suggested that this was due to exhaustion of the hypothalamus and/or the adrenal medulla. Death of 6 baboons was attributed to cardiovascular collapse owing to cardiac arrhythmias induced by hyperkalemia and acidosis. Correction of severe lactic acidosis may require administration of sodium bicarbonate. Hyperpyrexia can be treated with tepid sponging, cooling blankets, and antipyretic agents.

Myoglobinuria is occasionally seen in patients with SE and is indicative of severe muscle damage resulting from muscular activity, traumatic injury during seizures, and/or occluded regional blood supply and compressed muscle tissue from the mere weight of the body during coma.[25] Myoglobinuria is a major complication that may lead to renal failure, although only a few cases of prolonged tonic-clonic seizures leading to myoglobinuria renal failure have been reported.[25,26] In addition, marked myoglobinuria can occur without apparent alteration of renal function.[26]

DRUG TREATMENT OF SE

Diazepam

Diazepam (Valium®) is considered by many to be the drug of choice for the initial treatment of SE.[27–31] Intravenous diazepam is a fast-acting drug providing short-term control of seizure activity. In a review of studies on the use of diazepam in SE, Mattson[32] reported that while it was effective in stopping seizure activity, the duration of action was only 30–60 minutes.

Current evidence suggests that diazepam exerts its anticonvulsant activity by influencing the inhibitory neurotransmitter, GABA.[33] Reduction of GABA at neuronal receptor sites is known to enhance or elicit seizure activity.[34] Whether diazepam acts at the presynaptic or postsynaptic level to increase GABA is not entirely clear, nor is the exact molecular nature of the diazepam-neuronal interaction known.[33]

The recommended dosage of diazepam is 15–20 mg I.V. to be given at a rate of 5 mg or less per minute. Therapeutic plasma level is 0.5 mcg/ml or greater. When 20 mg of diazepam is administered I.V. over 10 minutes to a 70 kg man, the therapeutic level is maintained for 1–2 hours.[28] If diazepam is going to work, the effects are almost immediate and seizures will usually stop during the injection or within a few minutes of completing the injection. Although diazepam gives immediate control of seizures, its effects are not lasting thus necessitating the use of a longer-acting anticonvulsant, usually phenytoin or phenobarbital. An advantage of diazepam is that it controls seizures quickly and allows time for administration of maintenance drugs.

Diazepam is contraindicated in patients with glaucoma and those having known hypersensitivity to the drug. Adverse reactions include respiratory depression and hypotension; Bell[44] advised careful monitoring of the patient.

The effects are additive when used in conjunction with several depressant drugs, particularly phenobarbital. Because of its marked muscle relaxant effect, there is increased possibility of the tongue occluding the airway. Diazepam may produce a hypnotic effect and can reduce the level of consciousness even further in comatose patients. Less serious effects include ataxia, drowsiness, and diplopia.

An alternative to diazepam I.V. push is the infusion technique. A constant infusion of diazepam is advantageous since it allows the maintenance of a sustained high plasma diazepam level. Enrile-Bascal and Delgado-Escueta[36] found that infusion of diazepam at a rate of 8 mg/hr ensured a serum level of 0.2–0.4 mcg/ml. However, due to its cardiorespiratory depressant effect, careful monitoring of vital signs was advised. Dam and Christiansen[37] found that Valium® brand of diazepam precipitates in a dextrose solution and recommended that a nondextrose solution be used as a diluent. Parlar et al[38] also found that because diazepam appears to bind to the plastic in I.V. bags, its potency can be decreased. Since no reaction was found with glass, this was recommended as the container of choice if the infusion technique is to be used.

Phenytoin

Intravenous phenytoin sodium (Dilantin®) is also used for control of SE and exerts an anticonvulsant action that begins 10–20 minutes after infusion. Woodbury[39] concluded that the major effect of phenytoin is to decrease the intracellular influx of Na^+ and Ca^{++} and, in turn, block neurotransmitter release.

The recommended dose of phenytoin for SE is 12–18 mg/kg intravenously. Because phenytoin can cause cardiac dysrhythmias, it should be given no faster than 50 mg/min and the ECG should be monitored continuously. Phenytoin has a highly basic pH which causes it to crystallize readily in glucose solutions; this necessitates flushing the I.V. line with saline or alcohol prior to injection. A therapeutic plasma level of phenytoin is 10–20 mcg/ml. Maintenance doses average 300–400 mg/day. Phenytoin should not be administered I.M. because it precipitates in muscle tissue leading to slowed absorption,[40] and may cause local irritation and sterile abscesses.

Phenytoin is a popular drug for SE because of its long action. If given in adequate doses, the effects will last for 24 hours.[41] Because of its cardiotonic effects, phenytoin should be used with extreme caution, if at all, in patients with sinus bradycardia, sinoatrial block, second and third degree atrioventricular block, Stokes-Adams syndrome, hypotension, or severe myocardial insufficiency.[35] The drug is contraindicated in patients with a known hypersensitivity to phenytoin. Side effects most commonly occur when phenytoin is given too rapidly, and include hypotension, cardiac conduction disturbances, ventricular fibrillation, cardiovascular collapse, and respiratory arrest.[7] Rarely, myoclonic SE will occur with an excess of phenytoin. Wilder[45] studied the effectiveness of phenytoin in control of SE and concluded that it provided prompt therapeutic effects without masking cortical function.

Phenobarbital

Phenobarbital is commonly used for control of SE. The onset of action is 5–25 minutes. The most probable antiepileptic action is at the synapse. Barbiturates in general are known to increase the neuronal threshold to electrical and chemical stimuli, depress physiological excitation and enhance inhibition at the synapse (suggestive of an interaction with GABA), and reduce Ca^{++} uptake by depolarized nerve terminals (presumably reducing neurotransmitter release).[42] The exact mechanism of action specific for anticonvulsant therapy is unclear and may depend on the dose.[43] The recommended dose is 5–8 mg/kg of body weight, to be given at a rate no greater than 60 mg/min intravenously. The therapeutic plasma levels are 10–40 mcg/ml. The intramuscular route is not recommended for phenobarbital as it takes 1–2 hours to attain effective plasma levels. The maintenance dose in an adult is 60–300 mg/day. The advantage of phenobarbital is that it has a long duration of action (24 hours) similar to phenytoin. Phenobarbital is the drug of choice for barbiturate withdrawal SE. The side effects of phenobarbital include depression of respiration and consciousness, therefore caution should be exercized in using phenobarbital concurrently with other drugs such as diazepam, because the respiratory depressant effects may be additive.

The use of phenobarbital is contraindicated for patients who are hypersensitive to barbiturates and who have porphyria. Phenobarbital should be used with caution in patients with impaired respiratory, cardiac, renal, and hepatic function, myasthenia gravis, or myxedema. Toxic effects include sedation, cardiorespiratory depression, ataxia, drowsiness, and diplopia.[35] If a patient requires a larger dose of phenobarbital than 5–8 mg/kg to control SE, it is advisable to monitor the patient's respirations, heart rate, and blood pressure frequently. The patient may require intubation and assisted ventilation.

It is important for the nurse to understand that drugs used in the treatment of SE vary from physician to physician, depending on the individual's past experience and comfort in using a specific drug or combination of drugs.

ALTERNATIVE TREATMENTS

Refractory SE is a condition in which seizures do not respond to the usual anticonvulsant therapy. It is in this type of SE that most of the complications occur. Refractory SE can occur because precipitating factors were not or could not be treated, or because the dosages of anticonvulsant drugs were not adequate to reach or maintain a plasma concentration sufficient to stop the seizures. In these cases, the following drugs may be used: paraldehyde, neuromuscular blocking agents, general anesthesia, lidocaine.

Paraldehyde may be used when the patient fails to respond or is allergic to the first line drugs or if SE is due to alcohol withdrawal. It should be given I.V. or I.M. because absorption from the GI tract (via the nasogastric and rectal routes) is too slow. Intravenous paraldehyde should be diluted in normal saline to a 4% solution because higher concentrations can lead to precipitation of the drug in the veins. The recommended dose is 0.1–0.15 ml/kg to be repeated every 2–4 hours.[46] If paraldehyde comes in contact with plastic, it may produce toxic substances; therefore, glass containers should be used for parenteral administration. Intramuscular paraldehyde is very painful and can cause tissue necrosis and damage to nerves near the injection site. If the I.M. route is necessary, paraldehyde should be injected deep in the buttocks, taking care to avoid the sciatic nerve and to administer a maximum of only 5 ml per injection site.[35]

Neuromuscular blocking agents may be used to paralyze voluntary muscle when seizures become refractory. These drugs inhibit acetylcholine from binding to postsynaptic receptors at the neuromuscular junction, thus blocking impulse transmission. Complications of tonic-clonic activity (hyperthermia, myoglobinuria, and muscle damage) as well as physical injury may be prevented by paralyzing the patient. However, because respiratory muscles are also paralyzed, intubation and controlled ventilation are necessary. This form of paralysis does not prevent ongoing cerebral seizure activity, but offers the patient some relief from respiratory and circulatory demands resulting from excessive muscle activity, and allows for easier access to the patient for drug administration and maintenance of vital functions.

General anesthetics also prevent tonic-clonic movements and require artificial control of respirations. General anesthetics depress impulse conduction within the ascending reticular activating system (RAS). As the sensitivity or threshold to stimulation of the RAS is reduced, the activation of the cortex is reduced, suppressing the electrical activity of both the cortex and voluntary muscle.[47] Thus, general anesthesia reduces both cerebral seizure activity and cerebral metabolic needs. Presently there is no specific anesthetic consistently recommended, and the appropriate duration of treatment in SE has not been established. Since EEG and ECG monitoring is usually employed, a nonflammable anesthetic should be used.

Lidocaine hydrochloride, occasionally used to treat SE has been reported effective in stopping seizures when other drugs have failed.[46] It has not been approved for this use by the FDA, however, and therefore may not be routinely used. Knowledge of the action of lidocaine comes from studies of its antiarrhythmic effects on cardiac cells, where it decreases the permeability of the cell membrane to Na^+ and K^+, thereby increasing the threshold excitability. Fosher[35] recommended an initial I.V. bolus of 2–3 mg/kg with maintenance doses up to 3–10 mg/kg in refractory status. Since these recommendations far exceed the manufacturer's recommendations, constant monitoring of the patient's cardiovascular status is mandatory.

Sodium amobarbital I.V. may be used to treat SE although it has the disadvantage of causing frequent recurrence of seizures after the first episode has ceased. The rate of infusion is 50–100 mg/min, not to exceed 500 mg per dosage.[35] This drug is usually given by the physician because of its rapid onset of action and the risk of respiratory depression. The patient should be intubated, with a ventilator standing by if the seizures do not stop instantly and a large dose of the drug is required. Blood pressure should be monitored frequently since rapid I.V. administration may induce vasodilation and hypotension. For longer lasting control, sodium amobarbital may be followed with 100–300 mg of I.M. or I.V. phenobarbital.

Lorazepam is a benzodiazepine similar to diazepam. A study by Walker has shown it to be effective and safe treatment for SE[51] with little or no depressant effect on respiration or circulation. Serum concentrations remain at relatively high levels for at least 2 hours following I.V. injection. Further studies of lorazepam may demonstrate that it is preferable to diazepam, since it produces more sustained seizure control and has a reduced incidence of cardiorespiratory depression.

OTHER TYPES OF STATUS EPILEPTICUS

Epilepsia partialis continua is a form of focal motor status epilepticus. It may affect persons of all ages, and occurs in acute as well as chronic lesions of the brain. The clinical features are variable with each case. This disorder is characterized by irregular twitching of specific groups of skeletal muscles. It may appear to be a nonconvulsive type of movement disorder. Manifestations may vary initially but later may show an unchanging pattern. The response to anticonvulsant treatment is poor; intravenous diazepam has been used with short-term success. The prognosis for epilepsia partialis continua depends on the underlying disease. In a series of studies by Thomas and others,[53] the most common cause in children was a chronically progressive, possible inflammatory disease of the brain. In adults, focal cerebrovascular and neoplastic lesions were the most common causes. The prognosis varies with the cause.

Hypoglycemia leading to SE may occur occasionally. The patient is usually a known diabetic who has taken too much insulin. These attacks are characterized by a confused state followed by tonic-clonic seizures. Prior to the onset of the seizures, the patient may be able to identify that he is having a hypoglycemic attack. Treatment includes a bolus of 25–50 cc of 35–50% glucose solution. Frequent blood glucose levels should be drawn to evaluate the treatment.

ESTABLISHING A TREATMENT PROGRAM

To prevent SE from recurring, it is important to determine the precipitating cause. If the patient is a known epileptic, it must be determined if the cause was discontinuation of medications or abuse of other drugs such as barbiturates, alcohol, or tricyclic antidepressants. Plasma levels of these drugs should be checked. Drug absorption difficulties, metabolic changes, and structural lesions must also be considered. In any case of SE, the patient should have a complete neurological examination.

If the patient has never had a history of seizures, a complete seizure workup is required. A history of neurological and medical disorders, recent head injury, central nervous system (CNS) infection, or drugs and toxic substances should be sought. Laboratory tests as previously described should be thoroughly evaluated. An examination of cerebrospinal fluid should include glucose and protein, cell count and morphology, and a Gram's stain. A CT scan will identify intracranial bleeding, brain edema, tumors, and structural abnormalities of the brain. An EEG may be helpful after acute tonic-clonic SE to identify the specific seizure type.

After an episode of SE, the patient will usually be placed on a maintenance dose of one or more anticonvulsant drugs. The patient must understand why he or she is taking medication, when to take it, and the side effects. Many patients need encouragement to continue medications once their seizures have been controlled. They also must be aware that rapid withdrawal of anticonvulsants can cause SE.

SUMMARY

Tonic-clonic SE is a series of repetitive seizures lasting at least 30 minutes. It can be a symptom of an underlying structural brain lesion or a result of inadequate anticonvulsant medication intake in a known epileptic patient. Nurses must understand the etiology and pathogenesis of SE for proper care.

The most common and most life-threatening type of SE seen in the ICU is one that has become refractory to usual treatment methods. The patient usually requires extensive monitoring and maintenance of vital functions. Cardiovascular, respiratory, and central nervous system complications frequently occur due to refractory SE or side effects of therapy.

The three most commonly used anticonvulsants in treatment of tonic-clonic SE are diazepam, phenytoin, and phenobarbital. Often diazepam is used as the initial drug because of its fast onset of action. However, because it has a short duration, it should be followed by a longer-acting drug such as phenytoin or phenobarbital. Concurrent use of diazepam and phenobarbital may cause additive cardiorespiratory depressant effects and should be used with caution. Other drugs are implemented if the patient does not respond to firstline treatment. These include paraldehyde, neuromuscular blocking agents, and general anesthetics. Assisted ventilation and vigilant monitoring of vital functions is required with the latter two treatments because of motor paralysis.

Another type of SE, which is resistant to most therapy, is epilepsia partialis continua. This constant twitching of a part of the body may spontaneously cease or continue until the patient dies. Hypoglycemia may bring on SE characterized by a confused state followed by tonic-clonic seizures.

It is important for the nurse to assess neurological and cardiorespiratory function and to know the elements of the medical work-up on any patient who has had tonic-clonic SE. Since it is the nurse who gives the anticonvulsant drugs used for treatment of SE, she must know the onset and duration of their action as well as their side effects. The outcome of a patient with SE depends on diligent observation, safe and effective delivery of anticonvulsant medication, and proper maintenance of vital functions. These responsibilities present a great challenge to the critical care nurse.

ACKNOWLEDGMENTS

This paper was supported by NIH contract 1-NS-6-2431 National Institute of Neurological and Communicative Disorders and Stroke, PHS/DHHS, and grant ID-23-NU-00081-01, Division of Nursing, PHS/DHHS.

REFERENCES

1. Browne TR: Drug therapy review: drug therapy of status epilepticus. Am J Hosp Pharm 35:915–922, 1978.
2. Celesia GG: Modern concepts of status epilepticus, JAMA, 235:1571–1574, 1976.
3. Gastaut H: Clinical and electroencephalographical classification of epileptic seizures. Epilepsia (Suppl) 10:S2–S13, 1969.
4. Oxbury JM, Whitty CWM: Causes and consequences of status epilepticus in adults. Brain, 94:733–744, 1971.
5. Rowan AJ, Scott DF: Major status epilepticus. Acta Neurol Scand 46:573–584, 1970.
6. Simon RP, Aminoff MJ: Chemical aspects of status epilepticus in an unselected population. Ann Neurol 8:93, 1980.
7. Cranford RE, Leppik IE, Patrick B, et al: Intravenous phenytoin in acute treatment of seizures. Neurology 29:1474–1479, 1979.
8. Aicardi A, Chevrie JJ: Convulsive status epilepticus in infants and children. A study of 239 cases. Epilepsia 11:187–197, 1970.
9. Oppenheimer E and Rausman NP: Seizures in childhood: an approach to emergency management. Pediatr Clin North Am 26(4):837–854, 1979.
10. Solomon GE, Plum F: Clinical Management of Seizures: A Guide for the Physician. W.B. Saunders, Philadelphia, 1976.
11. Wyler A, Ward A: Epileptic neurons. In Lockard JS and Ward AA, Eds: Epilepsy: A Window to Brain Mechanisms. Raven Press, New York, (in press).
12. Meldrum B: Neuropathology and pathophysiology. pp. 331–336. In Laidlaw J and Richens A, Eds: A Textbook of Epilepsy, Churchill Livingstone, Edinburgh, 1976.
13. Meldrum B, Horton R: Physiology of status epilepticus in primates. Arch Neurol 28:1–9, 1973.
14. Chapman AG, Meldrum B, Siesjo BK: Cerebral metabolic changes during prolonged epileptic seizures in rats. J Neurochem 28:1025–1035, 1977.
15. Collins RD, Posner JB, Plum F: Cerebral energy metabolism during electroshock seizures in mice. Am J Physiol 218:943, 1970.
16. Noel P et al: Mesial temporal haemorrhage, consequence of status epilepticus. J Neurol Neurosurg Psychiatry 40:932–935, 1977.
17. Siesjo SK, Abdul-Kahman A: A metabolic basis for selective vulnerability of neurons in status epilepticus. Acta Physiol Scand 106:377–378, 1979.
18. Meldrum B: Physiological changes during prolonged seizures and epileptic brain damage. Neuropediatrie 9(3):203–212, 1978.

19. Meldrum B, Brierley JB: Prolonged epileptic seizures in primates. Arch Neurol 28:10–17, 1973.
20. Wasterlain CG, Plum F: Vulnerability of developing rat brain into electroconvulsive seizures. Arch Neurol 29:38–45, 1973.
21. Duffy FH, Lombroso CT: Treatment of status epilepticus. Clin Neuropharmacology 3:41–55, 1978.
22. Nicol C: Status epilepticus. JAMA 234(4):419–420, 1975.
23. Schneider S: Status epilepticus (letter). JAMA 235(18):1964, 1976.
24. Trubuhovich R: Management of severe or intractable convulsions including eclampsia. Int Anesthesiol Clin Summer–Fall:201–238, 1978.
25. Singahl PC, Chugh KS, Gulati DR: Myoglobinuria and renal failure after status epilepticus. Neurology 28:200–201, 1978.
26. Fischer S et al: Disseminated intravascular coagulation in status epilepticus. Thromb Haemost 38:909–913, 1977.
27. Duncan M: Status epilepticus in the child. p. 64. In Ferris G, Ed: Treatment of Epilepsy Today. Medical Economics, Oradell, N.J., 1978.
28. Gastaut H et al: Treatment of status epilepticus with diazepam. Epilepsia 6:167–182, 1965.
29. Richens A: Drug Treatment of Epilepsy. p. 98. Henry Kimpton, London, 1976.
30. Troupin A: The choice of anticonvulsants. p. 267. In Laidlaw J and Richens A, Eds: A Textbook of Epilepsy. Churchill-Livingston, Edinburgh, 1976.
31. Penry JK and Walter R: Summary and consensus on treatment of status epilepticus. Presented at the International Symposium on Status Epilepticus, Santa Monica, California. November 19, 1980.
32. Mattson R: The benzodiazepines. p. 497–518. In Woodbury, DM, Penry JK and Schmidt RP, Eds: Antiepileptic Drugs, Raven Press, New York, 1972.
33. Killam E, Saria A: Benzodiazepines. pp. 597–611. In Glaser GH, Penry JK, Woodbury PM, Eds: Antiepileptic Drugs: Mechanisms of Action. Raven Press, New York, 1980.
34. Haefly W, Kulcsar A, Mohler H et al: Possible involvement of GABA in the central actions of benzodiazepines. Adv Biochem Psychopharmacol 14:131–151, 1975.
35. Fosher W: Treatment of Status Epilepticus, University Park Press, Baltimore, 1979.
36. Enrile-Bascal F and Delgado-Escueta AV: IV diazepam in tonic-clonic status epilepticus. Presented at the International Symposium on Status Epilepticus, Santa Monica, California, November 19, 1980.
37. Dam M, Christiansen J: Diazepam: intravenous infusion in the treatment of status epilepticus. Acta Neurol Scand 54:278–280, 1976.
38. Parlar WA, Morris ME, Shearer CA: Incompatibility of diazepam injection in plastic intravenous bags. Am J Hosp Pharm 36:505–507, 1979.
39. Woodbury DM: Phenytoin: Proposed mechanisms of anticonvulsant action. pp. 447–471. In Glaser GH, Penry JK, Woodbury DM, Eds: Antiepileptic Drugs: Mechanisms of Action. Raven Press, New York, 1980.
40. Wilensky AJ and Lowden A: Inadequate serum levels after intramuscular administration of diphenylhydantoin. Neurology (Minneapolis) 23(3):318–324, 1973.
41. Cranford RE, Leppik I, Patrick B et al: Intravenous phenytoin: clinical and pharmacological aspects. Neurology 28:874–880, 1978.
42. Pritchard J: Phenobarbital: proposed mechanisms of antiepileptic action. In Glaser GH, Penry JK, Woodbury DM, Eds: Antiepileptic Drugs: Mechanisms of Action. Raven Press, New York, 1980.
43. Goldring J, Blaustein M: Barbiturates: Physiological effects II. p. 530. In Glaser

GH, Penry JK, Woodbury DM, Eds: Antiepileptic Drugs: Mechanisms of Action. Raven Press, New York, 1980.
44. Bell DS: Dangers of treatment of status epilepticus with diazepam. Br Med J 1:159–161, 1969.
45. Wilder BJ, Ramsey RE, Willmore LJ et al: Efficacy of intravenous phenytoin in the treatment of status epilepticus: kinetic of central nervous system penetration. Ann Neurol 1:511–518, 1977.
46. Browne T: Paradehyde, chlormethiazole, lidocaine. Presented at the International Symposium on Status Epilepticus, Santa Monica, California, November 19, 1980.
47. Meyers F, Jawetz E, Goldfin A: Review of Medical Pharmacology. p. 197. Lange Medical Productions, Los Altos, 1976.
48. Ritchie J, Greene W: Local anesthetics. pp. 302–303. In Goodman L, Gilman A, Eds: Pharmacological Basis of Therapeutics. Macmillan, New York, 1980.
49. Roland M, Thomson PD, Guichard A et al: Disposition kinetics of lidocaine in normal subjects. Ann NY Acad Sci 179:383–397, 1971.
50. Harrison D, Moltin P, Winkle R: Clinical pharmacokinetics of antiarrythmic drugs. Prog Cardiovasc Dis 20:3:217, 1977.
51. Walker JE, Homan RW, Vasko MR, et al: Lorazepam in status epilepticus. Ann Neurology 6:207–213, 1979.
52. Congdon P, Forsythe W: Intravenous clonazepam in the treatment of status epilepticus in children. Epilepsia 21:97–102, 1980.
53. Thomas J, Reagan T, Klass D: Epilepsia partialis continua. Arch Neurol 34(4):266, 1977.

8 | Central Nervous System Infections

Carol Salminen
Nancy Wanski

Infections of the central nervous system constitute a medical emergency. When CNS infection is suspected, immediate action should be taken to establish diagnosis, identify the causative agent, and institute appropriate therapy. Early diagnosis and treatment not only preserve life, but minimize serious neurological sequelae. Most central nervous system infections can be treated medically; however, some require surgical intervention for proper management. This chapter will deal with brain abscess, meningitis, epidural abscess, subdural empyema, infectious complications of intracranial monitoring, and infections associated with trauma and surgical procedures.

BRAIN ABSCESS

Brain abscess is defined as a localized collection of pus within the brain substance.[1] The majority of brain abscesses seen clinically are due to infections that occur elsewhere in the body and spread by one of several routes to brain tissue. Approximately half the infections that result in brain abscess arise from the middle ear, mastoid cells, or paranasal sinuses.[2] Infections from these foci may gain access to the brain in one of two ways. First, the bacteria may travel along the walls of the cerebral veins. An infection can enter the brain via diploic and emissary veins which traverse the bone, dura mater, subdural, and arachnoid spaces.[1,3-7] This method of bacterial migration can result in cerebral abscess formation in locations remote to the middle ear and nasal sinuses.[2]

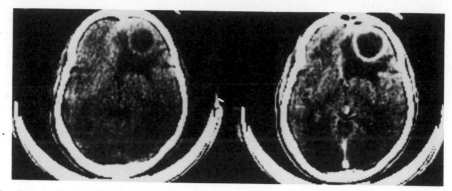

Fig. 8-1. An individual with brain abscess presented to the hospital with symptoms of severe headache, lethargy, rapidly progressing to coma. History revealed 2½ weeks earlier treatment for an abscessed tooth. (Left: unenhanced view; right: enhanced view)

The other route through which otogenic and rhinogenic infections may enter the brain is direct extension. An infection may form a tract that could actually erode through the cranial bone directly into the brain substance.[2] Infections of the middle ear or mastoid cells frequently result in temporal lobe abscess or less commonly in cerebella abscesses.[5,7–10] Cerebral abscesses that result from sinusitis commonly develop in the frontal and temporal lobes.[2]

The other major route of cerebral abscess formation is hematogenic and is, therefore, described as metastatic. The majority of these abscesses occur when septic emboli from the lungs or heart lodge in cerebral vessels and produce infection. Also, infections may spread from dental and peritonsillar abscess (Fig. 8-1), abdominal organs, or skin. These hematogenous infections tend to result in multiple abscess formation.[3,11]

Other less common causes of brain abscess include surgical intervention, trauma resulting in depressed or basilar skull fractures, and penetration of the cranial cavity by foreign bodies.[12–14] Meningitis rarely results in cerebral abscess.[2] In as many as 20% of the cases of cerebral abscess, no evidence of prior infection or trauma may be found.[5,15] A cerebral abscess begins as an inflammatory reaction that surrounds a focus of infection. Within a few days, the inflammatory process produces a central area of pus from liquification of necrotic tissue. Localized vascular congestion occurs and the surrounding brain tissue becomes edematous.[4,16–18] This initial inflammatory process is described as "cerebritis" and is seen on CAT scan as a region of decreased attenuation with poorly defined margins (Fig. 8-2A).[4,16–18] Spread of this suppurative process tends to occur by coalescense of adjacent tissue. Within a few days, fibroblasts migrate to the infection site and surround the purulent area with granulation tissue. (Fig. 8-2B).[4,16–18] As the process continues, fibroblastic activity and gliosis results in replacement of the granulation tissue by collagenous connective tissue. Encapsulation typically occurs within 2 weeks. (Fig. 8-2C).[4,16–18]

Cerebral abscesses of this nature may spread, producing satellite abscesses or abscesses in chains. The fibrous capsule as seen in Fig. 2C is frequently thinner at its deepest portions or not fully formed. This factor, along with the tendency of more distant vessels to become occluded from inflammation and edema, can result in spread of the abscess.[2]

The clinical course of brain abscess is remarkable because of its variation and unpredictability among individual patients. Many patients will have a relatively benign illness, while others will have rapid onset of symptoms, an abrupt downhill course, and will die in less than 10 days.[2] Severe headache is the most common initial symptom and is present in 70-90% of patients.[1,4,6] Other presenting signs may include lethargy, irritability, confusion, and coma.[1,4,6] Focal or generalized seizures will be present in one-third of patients.[11,19] Localizing neurological symptoms may develop and will vary according to abscess location. In 50% of the patients with cerebral abscess, an initial fever and leukocytosis will be present.[11,19] Frequently, a history of a recent exacerbation of infection will be obtained from those patients with chronic otitis, sinusitis, and pulmonary infections. Others may have a recent history of generally poor health.[3]

Cerebral abscess is associated with a 30–60% mortality rate.[1,4–6,20,21] One-half of those who survive the infection have neurological deficits which are often severe and incapacitating.[20,21] Early diagnosis is essential to avoid significant clinical deterioration and to allow for institution of appropriate therapy. Diagnostic studies may include lumbar puncture, electroencephalogram, brain scanning, arteriography and computerized axial tomography.[19]

In a study of 22 patients with brain abscess, Samson and Clark found that

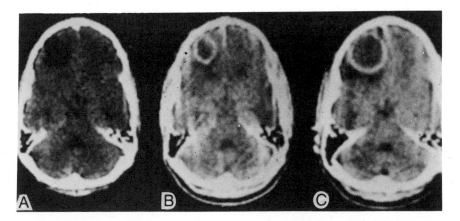

Fig. 8-2. Abscess formation: its three stages. (A) Cerebritis manifested by a region of decreased attenuation with poorly defined margins. (B) Vascular congestion: cerebral softening, note margin of abscess is more defined with the appearance of granulation tissue. (C) Mature capsule: thick capsule formation defined by fibrous tissue formation and gliosis.

although the cerebrospinal fluid was abnormal in the majority of the cases, it was completely normal in 4 patients.[22] Expected CSF findings include a slight increase in pressure, white cell count, and protein measurements.[5,6,20,21] The glucose should be normal and cultures should be sterile, unless the abscess is accompanied by meningitis.[5,22,23] It must be remembered that performing lumbar puncture on patients with increased intracranial pressure can result in shifting of brain tissues, brainstem compression, and death.[5,6,20-22] Therefore, in patients with indications of elevation in intracranial pressure, the diagnosis should be made without the assistance of lumbar puncture.

The electroencephalogram (EEG) is useful in approximately 50% of brain abscesses for localizing the lesion.[5,23] The EEG may show an area of high voltage slow wavy activity or phase reversal and electrical silence in the area of the abscess.[4]

Abscesses of 1 centimeter or more are easily demonstrable on brainscan using radioactive technetium (Fig. 8-3).[4,5] Brain scanning is particularly useful in diagnosing multiple abscesses.[24] Cerebral arteriography has been useful in diagnosing brain abscess, but is of limited value prior to abscess encapsulation. Also, with angiography brain abscess may be confused with metastatic tumor because of a ring stain that may be present in both.[4,5] Additionally, angiography, being an invasive procedure, is associated with some degree of morbidity.[4,5]

Currently, the most accurate tool available for the identification and localization of brain abscess is computerized axial tomography (CAT). Brain abscess is detected on CAT scan by localized changes in brain density caused by the infection.[25] These changes in density can be accentuated by an intravenous injection of contrast material.[25] Additionally, CAT scanning can differentiate between the cerebritis and encapsulation stages of brain abscess, the latter of which has implications for therapy (Fig. 8-2).[25]

Despite the diagnostic tools at our disposal, diagnosis of brain abscess frequently is not considered until the patient's neurological status has markedly deteriorated. Because recovery is closely related to the clinical status of the patient at the time the abscess is discovered and therapy instituted, diagnosis should not be delayed.[5,6,9]

Controversy exists over whether cerebral abscess should be treated with antibiotic therapy alone or antibiotic therapy in combination with surgical drainage or excision. Typically, the therapeutic regimen chosen depends upon a number of factors: the site of the abscess, the stage of development, and the causative organism. If an abscess is diagnosed early in the cerebritis stage, in many cases it can be cured with antibiotics.[21] Antibiotics instituted at this time will be started without the benefit of Gram's stain or culture, and instead are presecribed according to abscess location.[5] If the abscess is located in the frontal lobe, streptococcus is considered to be the most likely causative organism and penicillin is the drug of choice. Abscesses located in the temporal or cerebellar areas and metastatic abscesses are frequently of mixed flora and should be treated with a combination of antibiotics that include penicillin, ampicillin, metronidazole, chloramphenicol, or gentamicin.[6] When adminis-

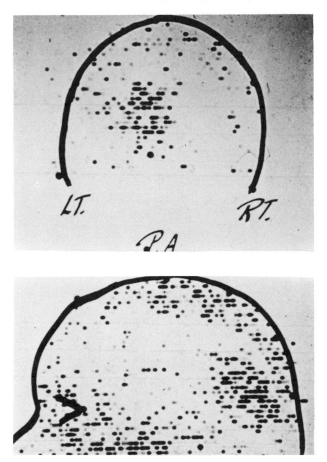

Fig. 8-3. Brain scan showing posteroanterior and left lateral views defining and abscess in the occipital lobe. (Fiengold SM: Central nervous system infection. pp 155–164. In Finegold S Ed: Anaerobic Infections. Academic Press, New York, 1978)

tering antibiotics in this situation, the effect of the blood-brain-barrier on absorption of the drug into the cerebrospinal fluid should be considered.[26] To obtain adequate levels of antibiotic in the CSF, the drug may be administered intrathecally by means of a ventriculostomy or may be injected directly into the abscess after surgical aspiration or drainage.

Elevation of intracranial pressure at this stage of therapy should be treated in the customary manner. Prompt and continued improvement should be expected after institution of antibiotic therapy and control of intracranial hypertension. If this does not occur, then surgical intervention with aspiration of the abscess for the purpose of positive organism identification and drainage should be performed.[5,23] Surgical drainage with or without total resection is indicated in patients treated medically who develop persistent increased intracranial pressure and in those patients who intially present with a fully developed, encapsulated abscess.[2,5] All patients should be placed on antimicrobial therapy for 3–4 weeks.[5,15] Glucocorticoids are often prescribed in addition to antimicrobial therapy.[5]

Proper management of cerebral abscess includes treatment of the primary infection to prevent the possibility of repeat abscess formation.[5,15] Successful treatment depends upon early diagnosis, accurate localization, and prompt institution of therapy. Nurses should be alert to the development of the signs and symptoms of cerebral abscess when caring for a patient with a recent history of ear or sinus infection. Brain abscess should be suspected in patients with bacterial endocarditis, lung infections, or acute abdominal infections who develop alterations in mental status or signs of localizing disease. For patients diagnosed with brain abscess, a thorough and ongoing neurological assessment should be done to aid in localization of lesion, detection of increased intracranial pressure, and, imminent herniation. Indicated nursing interventions for increased intracranial pressure, seizures, and postcraniotomy status should be carried out. Patients undergoing therapy should be closely monitored to ascertain their response to medical and surgical interventions. Patient and family support through this critical illness will be necessary. Families should understand that the mortality rate in cerebral abscess is high and that there is a possibility of permanent neurological deficiency with survival.

SUBDURAL EMPYEMA

Subdural empyema is a suppurative process that occurs between the dura and the outer surface of the arachnoid. Micro-organisms enter the area either by way of the emissary veins or as an extension of an osteomyelitic process. Subdural empyema occurs four times more frequently in males than females for unknown reasons.[27,28] Pus may be found over one or both hemispheres, the base of the brain, or along the falx cerebri.[29] Infection extends from the paranasal sinuses in 50% of patients with subdural empyema. The middle ear and mastoid area are implicated in 10–20% of cases. Other causative conditions include: trauma, surgical procedures, and preexisting subdural hematoma.[30]

Subdural empyema evolves rapidly. Presenting symptoms are fever, focal headaches which become generalized as the infection progresses, vomiting, and other signs of meningeal irritation.[27,31,32] Alteration in mental status is accompanied by focal or generalized seizures in half of the patients. If treatment is not instituted early following presentation of these symptoms, increased intracranial pressure, coma, and eventual tentorial herniation can be expected to occur.

Computerized axial tomography (CAT scan) is considered the most accurate diagnostic tool. The empyema can be seen as a zone of low attenuation representing pus, over the surface of the brain.[17] Significant cerebrospinal fluid findings include an elevation in pressure and an increase in neutrophils. (Table 8-1) This differs from the CSF findings in the patient with brain abscess.

Recommended treatment is surgical drainage by craniotomy or burrholes with subsequent irrigation of the subdural space.[28,33] Appropriate antibiotic

Table 8-1. Cerebrospinal fluid characteristics on the various central nervous system infections

Type of infectious process	Gross appearance	Cells	Cell types	Protein	Glucose	Gram's stain/ Culture
Bacterial meningitis	Turbid	High	Predominantly polymorpho-nuclear	Increased	Decreased, occasion-ally normal	Organisms isolated easily on culture, positive Gram's stain on 50% of patients
Viral meningitis	Clear, may be turbid	Low	Predominantly monocytes, early polymorpho-nuclear leukocytosis	Slightly increased	Normal	Echo virus 9 may be isolated, others less often
Tuberculous meningitis	Clear	Low	Predominantly monocytes	Increased	Normal early, decreased later	Cultures usually positive, occasionally seen on Gram's stain
Brain abscess	Clear	Low.	Predominantly lymphocytes	Increased	Normal	Nonspecific, unless abscess has ruptured into the ventricles
Subdural empyema		High	Predominantly neutrophils	Increased	Normal	Sterile
Epidural abscess	Clear	Low	Occasionally lymphocytes and neutrophils	Slightly increased		

therapy is prescribed according to the site of primary infection, and may be altered when microbiological results are available.[30] Bacterial organisms most often incriminated in subdural empyema include streptococci, staphlococci, various gram-negative organisms, aerobic and microaerophilic streptococci, and *Bacteroides fragilis*.[27,28,30]

In patients who receive prompt treatment, there is a good potential for complete neurological recovery. With subdural empyema, as with the brain abscess, morbidity and mortality are closely tied to the clinical status of the patient at the time therapy is instituted.

EPIDURAL ABSCESS

Epidural abscess is a suppurative process almost always associated with a focal area of osteomyelitis.[34] The area of infection is usually sharply defined and leads to a localized stripping of the periosteal dura (the outer-most layer of dura covering the brain) from cranial bone.[7,31,34] Subdural empyema often accompanies the epidural infection due to the ease with which the bacteria traverse the dura via emissary veins.[34]

Presenting symptoms include local pain, a generalized headache accompanied at times by an alteration of mental status, and seizures. With enlargement of the abscess, papilledema and other manifestations of intracranial hypertension may develop.[34] If the infection remains untreated and is allowed to extend, rapid neurological deterioration results.

Epidural abscess is easily detectable by CAT scan.[17,35,36] Recommended treatment includes surgical drainage and broad spectrum antibiotic coverage.[27,28,30,34] Cerebrospinal fluid for Gram's stain, culture, and sensitivity should be obtained. Antimicrobial therapy should be modified, if indicated, when results become available.[34]

MENINGITIS

Meningitis should be upermost in the minds of health care personnel when a patient presents with fever, nausea, vomiting, recent mental derangement, and neurological symptoms. A diagnosis of meningitis becomes more likely if these symptoms are accompanied by a history of head trauma or recent infections. As meningitis is a life-threatening pyogenic infection, it is necessary to confirm the diagnosis early and promptly institute antimicrobial and/or supportive therapy.[37]

Early meningitis may resemble influenza with a low-grade fever, headache, and minimal nuchal pain and stiffness.[21,38] Although most patients show changes in mental function when first seen, some may be alert or only mildly lethargic.[21] Other common symptoms exhibited in the adult and older child include progressive headache, lethargy, stupor, seizures, nuchal rigidity, and occasionally pain. As the disease progresses, coma and neurological deficits may develop. (Table 8-2).[37-41] Some patients with bacterial meningitis will present in a deteriorated neurological condition and in septic shock. Initial management in these cases should include prompt administration of fluids, mechanical ventilation if indicated, and treatment of the bacterial infection.[42]

Cerebrospinal fluid examination is currently the most valuable tool available for diagnosing meningitis. Most often, the diagnosis can be established based upon typical CSF findings in combination with the clinical presentation. Once a specimen has been obtained, it must be transported immediately to the laboratory, since some causative organisms are fastidious with complex nutritional requirements and require prompt plating on appropriate agar.[21] Laboratory testing should include cultures, a total and differential cell count, and

Table 8-2. Common clinical findings in meningitis

Infection	Meningeal irritation	Mental function	Neurological abnormalities
Fever (100–106°F)	Headache	Lethargy	Seizures
Tachycardia	Nuchal rigidity	Confusion	Cranial nerve palsies
Chills	Stiff back	Delirium	Hemiparesis
Skin rash	Brudzinki's sign	Stupor	Hemiplegia
	Kernig's sign	Coma	Other focal neurologic signs

Table 8-3. Specific antimicrobial therapy for meningitis

Organism cultured	Drug of choice	Alternative therapy
Staphlococcus aureus	Nafcillin Loading dose 50 mg/kg I.V. in first hour. Maintenance dose 200 mg/kg/day I. V.	Vancomycin: 7.0 mg/kg/day or Erythromycin: Loading dose 15 mg/kg I.V. in first 30 minutes. Maintenance dose 75 mg/kg/day I.V.
E. coli, Proteus, Enterobacter cloacae, Klebsiella, Serratia, Citrobacter, Providencia	Ampicillin Loading dose 50 mg/kg hour. Maintenance dose 400 mg/kg/day I.V. Carbenicillin: Loading dose 100 mg/kg I.V. in first hour. Maintenance dose 300 mg/kg/day I.V.	Amikacin 7.5 mg/kg initially in first hour then 7.5 mg/kg q 12 hours. Gentamicin 1.5 mg/kg in first hour. Maintenance dose 3–5 mg/kg/day. Doses should be adjusted in both Amikacin and Gentamicin in patients with renal impairment.
Pseudomonas	Carbenicillin Loading dose 100 mg/kg I.V. in first hour. Maintenance dose 300–500 mg/kg/day I.V. Gentamicin Loading dose 1.5 mg/kg I.V. in first hour. Maintenance dose 3–5 mg/kg/day I.V. Intrathecal administration may be necessary in order to achieve adequate CSF levels. Intrathecal dose is 4 mg q 12 hours.	Amikacin 15 mg/kg/day I.V.
Streptococcus pneumoniae	Ampicillin 200–400 mg/kg/day I.V. Penicillin G 250,000 units/kg/day I.V. in children 2 months. In adults 15–20 million units/day, I.V. divided in 6–8 doses.	Chloramphenicol: Pediatric dose— 50–100 mg/kg/day I.V. Adult dose Loading dose 25 mg/kg initially in first hour. Maintenance dose 25–100 mg/kg/day I.V.
H. influenzae	Ampicillin 200–400 mg/kg/day. Loading dose 50 mg/kg I.V. in first hour.	Chloramphenicol Loading dose 25 mg/kg initially I.V. in first hour. Maintenance dose 25–100 mg/kg/day I.V.
N. meningititidis	Penicillin G Adults 15–20 million units/day I.V. Pediatric 250,000 units/kg/day. Ampicillin Loading dose 50 mg/kg I.V. in first hour. Maintenance dose 200–400 mg/kg/day I.V.	Chloramphenicol: Pediatric 50–100 mg/kg/day I.V. Adult 25–100 mg/kg/day I.V. Crystalline penicillin G 50,000 units/kg/day I.V. q 4 hours.
Mycobacterium tuberculosis	Isoniazid Pediatric dose 15 mg/kg/day I.M. or P.O. Adult dose 300 mg I.M. or P.O. per day. Streptomycin 20 mg/kg/day I.M./day. Para-aminosalicylic acid 150 mg/kg/day.	Ethambutal 25 mg/kg/day P.O. Rifampin Pediatric dose 5–10 mg/kg/day. Adult 600 mg/day P.O.
Anaerobic organisms	Chloramphenicol Loading dose 25 mg/kg I.V. initially in first hour. Maintenance dose 25–100 mg/kg/day I.V.	Penicillin G 250,000 units/kg/day I.V. in children 2 months of age. Adults 20–25 million units/day in divided doses.

References: 15, 20, 21, 26, 32, 37, 38, 39, 40, 44, 45, 46.

measurement of protein and glucose concentrations. A Gram's stain of the sediment of centrifuged spinal fluid should be done to provide basis for antimicrobial therapy.[37] A WBC count in excess of 1000/cu mm, and elevated protein level, and a glucose less than 50% of the serum glucose are consistent with meningitis. Blood specimens drawn for culture and sensitivity are positive in over one-half of patients. Other tests that may be ordered include serologic studies to define presence of fungus or virus, and counterimmunoelectrophoresis for bacterial antigens to detect meningococcal organisms, pneumococcus, or Hemophilus influenzae in CSF.[43]

Once the diagnosis is confirmed, the antimicrobial therapy should be as specific as possible. Antibiotics will be initiated on the basis of the patient's clinical condition, specimen Gram stains, patient age, epidemiologic factors, and the presence of underlying disease.[37–39,43] The intravenous route of antibiotic administration is preferred. Once the causative organism is identified and the sensitivity is available, antibiotic therapy can be adjusted if necessary. Recommended antimicrobial regimens are sbown in Table 8-3.

BACTERIAL MENINGITIS

The growth of bacteria in and adjacent to the leptomeninges (the pia and arachnoid membranes) and the cerebrospinal fluid constitutes bacterial meningitis. Since the subarchnoid space extends over the entire brain and spinal cord, infection at any location rapidly moves throughout the entire space and into the ventricles. Bacteria that produce the infection generate a thick exudate that results in viscous CSF.[13] Normal flow and absorption may be interrupted, which contributes to an increase in intracranial pressure.[13] During meningitis, cerebral edema is always present although the exact cause is not clear.[13] Additionally, the infection results in a disturbance of normal cerebral functioning, which accounts for the frequently altered level of consciousness and other neurologic deficits. The exact mechanism responsible for these findings has not been delineated.[3,13] Exudate is frequently present over the base of the brain, and over the sheaths of cranial and spinal nerves.[2]

The majority of cases of bacterial meningitis are caused by either *Hemophilus influenzae, Streptococcus pneumoniae*, or *Neisseria meningitidis*.[13] However, some studies have shown *Klebsiella, E. coli, Staphlococcus aureus*, and *Pseudomonas aeruginosa* to be frequent causes of meningitis.[47] The causative bacteria are frequently from the patient's own endogenous flora, either normal or altered by antibiotic treatment and exposure. Organisms evidently reach the meninges via the bloodstream. Predisposing conditions to the development of bacterial meningitis are otitis media, mastoiditis, sinusitis, tonsillitis, sepsis, and pleuropulmonary infections. Contamination of the meninges can occur due to penetrating head trauma, surgery, catheter implantation, or as a result of cerebral abscess rupture into a ventricle.[23] Nonpenetrating head injuries frequently lead to staphlococcal, streptococcal gram-negative meningeal infections.[21] Meningitis resulting from trauma does not always occur immediately but may develop years later. Delayed meningeal infections are usually the result of dural tears associated with fistula information.[21] Thus, the history of both recent and remote trauma can be extremely important in diagnosing the cause of meningitis.

Two-thirds of the cases of bacterial meningitis occur in children, usually under the age of 5.[38,44] Exact cause of death in bacterial meningitis is frequently unclear, but may relate to causes other than meningitis itself. The mortality rate ranges from 10-30% and is highest in neonates.[13] Fever and dehydration secondary to decreased oral intake and emesis predispose patients to seizures.[40]

Supportive therapy in the form of maintenance of patent airway, assisted ventilation, and correction of fluid and electrolyte imbalances may become necessary.[20] Attention should be given to adequate oxygenation and cardiac monitoring. For antibiotic therapy,[42] see Table 8-3.

MENINGOCOCCAL MENINGITIS

Meningococcal meningitis, caused by the bacterium *Neisseria meningitidis*, is considered one of the most contagious forms of meningitis and is associated with a high mortality in its fulminant form. It is worldwide in its distribution and occurs in sporadic and epidemic forms; therefore, it deserves special mention. While all age ranges may be affected, males contract the infection twice as often as females. No apparent racial susceptibility or immunity exists.[38] There have been epidemics of meningococcal meningitis in the past, coinciding with wartime and major population movements but none has occurred in this country since World War II.[13] *N. meningitidis* first appears in the nasopharynx and can remain viable there for weeks unless cultured and appropriate antimicrobial therapy presecribed. The bacteria enter the bloodstream, from the nasopharynx, produce septicemia and can result in metastatic infections in all organs including the meninges.[13] While the organism is transmissable to others by intimate contact or droplet spread, indirect transmission is highly unlikely because of the vulnerability of the organism to heat and drying.[38,42]

The incubation period is from 2–10 days and the actual infection process is divided into three phases: local or nasopharyngeal, invasive or septicemic and meningeal. The local or nasopharyngeal phase is usually subclinical but may present with nonspecific respiratory complaints. This phase is defined only if nasopharyngeal cultures are taken.[37,38] During the invasive or septicemic phase bacteria enter the blood stream and fever, chill, muscle aches, and hypotension occur. A petechial rash, the hallmark of the disease, will be present in approximately 65% of the cases. The rash first appears on the ankles and wrists in older children and adults and later involves the trunk but is generalized in infants and younger children. Lesions range in size from 1 millimeter to 1 centimeter and may become hemorrhagic. Large ecchymotic or purpuric lesions are present predominantly on the face and extremities in the fulminant form of the disease. By careful scrapping of the lesion with a scalpel blade, followed by a gram stain of the fluid obtained, *N. meningitidis* may be isolated.[13,37,38,42] This phase can persist for weeks or months in chronic meningococcemia with recurrent fever, chills joint pain and petechial lesions.[38] During the meningeal phase, inflammation of the meninges occurs due to invasion of the organism along with fever, chills, severe throbbing headache, vomiting, and nuchal rigidity. The development of the symptoms may be insidious or abrupt. Other complications may include septic shock and vascular collapse.[13] Specific therapy is essential to prevent prolonged morbidity and significant mortality.[38,40,44] Penicillin is the drug of choice and Rifampin for those individuals with a penicillin allergy. (see Table 8-3 for appropriate dosages and schedules.

Patients should be considered most contagious during the acute phase of the infection, even though they are capable of spread during the nasopharyngeal phase. Strict isolation procedures should be instituted and maintained until at least 24 hours after institution of appropriate antibiotics.[23,37-39,40,44] All secretions should be handled carefully even though the organism is susceptible to heat and drying. After 24 of antimicrobial therapy isolation procedures may be discontinued.[34-36,38,40,41] Prophylaxis is not necessary for hospital contacts among nursing personnel, etc, unless the isolation procedures were not followed and gross breaks in technique occurred.[38]

VIRAL MENINGITIS

Viral meningitis occurs almost uniformly as a complication of a primary viral infection outside the central nervous system.[2] Among the most common etiologic agents are enteroviruses, mumps virus, herpes, and arboviruses.[41] Viruses are transmitted by multiple routes, but the most frequent methods of infestation are the oral, fecal-oral, or respiratory pathways.[37,41] Children and young adults are at greatest risk for development of viral meningitis. Once the virus enters the body it replicates, produces generalized viremia, and spreads to the CNS, usually by a hematogenous route.[41] The cerebrospinal fluid is usually clear but may be slightly turbid. An early predominance of neutrophils will be replaced by mononuclear cells within 48 hours of the onset (Table 8-1).[37,38,41]

Different viruses appear to have variable affinity for certain structures within the CNS. Signs and symptoms manifested tend to reflect those structures affected by the virus.[41] Onset of illness is usually quite sudden and may be characterized by intense frontal or periorbital headache, undulant fevers, Kernig's and Brudzinki's signs, malaise, drowsiness, tinnitus, vertigo, nausea, vomiting, nuchal rigidity, and pain in the chest and abdomen.[41]

Treatment consists of bedrest, isolation during febrile period, analgesic drugs, and correction of fluid and electrolyte imbalance, if present.[41] The recovery period can be expected to vary from a few days to several weeks.[37,38] Meningitis caused by enterovirus is known to result in neuromuscular paralytic effects, therefore, activity during convalescence must be graded for these patients.[41,42] Residual weakness following recovery may be present and must be watched for.[41]

ANAEROBIC MENINGITIS

Compared to bacterial or viral meningitis, anaerobic bacterial meningitis occurs frequently. It is usually found in association with a more extensive intracranial infection.[15,46] Common sources of anaerobic meningitis include cerebral abscess rupture, sinusitis, pharyngitis, otitis media, and surgical procedures such as craniotomy and laminectomy. Head trauma resulting in open skull fractures, severe scalp lacerations. or dural tears may allow anaerobic organisms to contaminate the meninges.[32,48]

The symptomology and clinical course of anaerobic meningitis is consistent with other types of meningitis. Antibiotic therapy is often the same as for other forms of bacterial meningitis. See Table 8-3 for recommended drugs and dosages.

TUBERCULOUS MENINGITIS

Tuberculous meningitis is caused by the acid-fast bacterium *Mycobacterium tuberculosis*. It has a low occurrence rate in the United States. It affects all age groups, but more commonly, in children.[2] In most patients, there will be evidence of a concurrent, active tuberculosis infection elsewhere in the body.[2] Signs and symptoms usually develop slowly and include weight loss, listlessness, headache, emesis, drowsiness, photophobia, and nuchal rigidity.[45] The characteristic presence of fever and cranial nerve palsies in association with other symptoms should make one suspicious of TB meningitis.[21,45] CSF examination may not be helpful in making the diagnosis. Studies have shown smears to be positive in only 10% of patients while cultures yielded the organism in between 40-90% of patients.[45]

Appropriate pharmacologic intervention consists of triple therapy: isoniazid (INH), streptomycin, and paraaminosalicyclic acid (PAS). Alternative drug therapy would include INH, ethambutal, and/or rifampin.[21] Drug therapy should be continued for 2 years.

The mortality ranges between 15–35% of those patients with serious disease.[43] Unless pulmonary tuberculosis is also present, isolation procedures are not indicated. Refer to Tables 8-2 and 8-3 for the CSF findings and antimicrobial regimen.

INFECTIONS ASSOCIATED WITH TRAUMA
AND SURGICAL PROCEDURES

Mechanisms leading to bacterial infection of the CNS due to trauma have been discussed elsewhere in this chapter. Therefore, discussion here will be confined to scalp lacerations and blunt trauma.

Every scalp laceration should be regarded as a potential source of infection. Improper management of a scalp laceration can result in a subgaleal, epidural, or subdural abscess.[49] Bacterial meningitis can develop from a penetrating injury (see bacterial meningitis). Certain principles should be followed in the care of lacerations: 1) all scalp lacerations should be thoroughly examined; 2) hair should be shaved around the laceration; 3) the wound and subgaleal space, if penetrated, should be irrigated using sterile technique with copious amounts of sterile saline or antibiotic solution; 4) irrigation should be followed with application of a sterile surgical dressing.[49,50] If the skin has been severely traumatized, or the wound was heavily soiled by foreign matter, antibiotics should be given for a period of 5 days; one of the cephalothins is ususally chosen.

Blunt trauma without cranial penetration can also result in infection. Organisms presumably enter from the oropharynx via a recognized or occult skull fracture.[21] In simple fractures, the fracture itself does not lead to infection. Rather, it is the exudate within the fracture that clots and occludes the break that provides an excellent medium for the growth of bacteria.[21] In patients who develop meningitis following nonpenetrating injuries, streptococcus pneumoniae is by far the most common cause.[21,40] Meningitis due to trauma can occur years after the traumatic event secondary to a tear in the dura and subsequent development of a cerebrospinal fluid fistula.[21,38] Anytime the cranial cavity or spinal canal is interrupted, it is susceptible to possible infection. Infection may occur at the time of the operative procedure or invasive procedure, or during the healing process. Factors contributing to the development of craniotomy and laminectomy wound infections include reexploration, lengthy operation, the use of external drains or monitoring devices, foreign penetration, and the patient's clinical condition at the time of the operation.[51-53] The incidence of infection associated with surgical procedures varies between 3–7%.[51,52] Serious morbidity and mortality figures may be as high as 20%.[52]

Nursing interventions should be directed toward prevention and detection of infections. Proper wound management includes maintenance of a dry encompassing sterile dressing which should be changed if it becomes wet. Only closed drainage systems should be utilized in these patients. Drains should be emptied at regular intervals, with attention to prevention of bacterial contamination. Indications of infection revealed in the laboratory data, vital signs, or neurological assessment should be reported immediately.

INFECTIOUS COMPLICATIONS ASSOCIATED WITH INTRACRANIAL PRESSURE MONITORING

Continuous intracranial pressure monitoring now plays a significant role in the management of the neurosurgical patient. Along with the innovation of these devices, however, is the possibility of serious infection that may result from their use.

The incidence of infectious complications in patients with intracranial monitoring devices reportedly ranges between 2–18%.[54,55] Incidence of infectious complications appears to closely parallel the duration of monitoring.[54,55] Complications reported in association with intracranial monitoring include meningitis, catheter site infections, ventriculitis, positive CSF cultures, and fistula formation.[54,55] Infections of this nature prolong hospitalization and significantly increase mortality.[55] Mortality rates for patients with infections have been reported to be as high as 70% compared to 33% in monitored patients without infectious complications.[55] While the use of prophylactic antibiotics to reduce incidence of intracranial infections is considered to be of no value, early discontinuation of monitoring devices can greatly diminish infections.[55]

In our Neurosurgical Intensive Care Unit, intraventricular monitoring is used almost exclusively. We find this method to be superior as it allows for measurement of intracranial pressure, controlled drainage of CSF, sampling of fluid for culture, and a means of administering medication. In an effort to avoid possible bacterial contamination and subsequent complications, the following stringent infection control measures have been instituted by our staff:

1. Development of a one piece, closed drainage unit for our patients with ventriculostomy who require drainage. The tubing and drainage unit are one complete unit inclusive of drip chamber with leur-lock connections. The drainage unit is changed every 24 hours.

2. Stringent sterile technique is followed with assembly of the monitoring devices and tubing, as well as during catheter placement. This includes both sterile glove and sterile field.

3. If the intraventricular catheter is required for longer than 72 hours, it is removed and another catheter is inserted into the opposite ventricle.

4. All CSF samples are drawn utilizing sterile technique at the stopcock-catheter junction. The procedure is taught to all nurses, residents, and interns to insure understanding and proper performance of sampling.

5. Whenever a dead head is removed from the system, a new sterile dead head is applied.

6. A dry sterile dressing is placed over and around the catheter insertion site. The dressing is checked frequently to detect leakage.

Prior to the institution of the above measures, we experienced a low incidence of meningitis, venticulitis, and insertion site infections. The most frequently encountered organisms were *Acinetobacter, Enterobacter, Staphlococcus epidermidis, Staphlococcus aureus, Streptococcus*, and *Pseudomonas*. With these procedures and the cooperation of physicians and nursing personnel, we hope to see a reduction in our already low incidence of infectious complications. We are confident that our high level of patient care results in minimal complications from invasive procedures.

REFERENCES

1. Meyer D; Brain abscess. pp 780–785. In Mandell GL, Douglas RG Jr, Eds. Principles and Practices of Infectious Diseases. John Wiley and Sons, New York, 1979
2. Adams D, Maurice Victor: Principles of Neurology. pp. 618–653. McGraw-Hill, New York, 1977
3. Raimondi AJ, Wright RL: Cranial and intracranial infections. pp 1547–1555. In Youmans J, Ed: Neurological Survey, a Comprehensive Reference Guide to the

Diagnosis and Management of Neurosurgical Problems. Vol. 3 WB Saunders, Philadelphia, 1973

4. Hendley JO: Brain abscess. pp 47–53. In Hook E, Mandell G, Gwaltney JM Jr, Sande MA Eds.: Current Concepts of Infectious Disease. John Wiley and Sons, New York, 1977

5. Weiss Martin: CNS infection, surgical intervention. LAC-USC Medical Center CD Grand Rounds. August 1980

6. Garfield J: Management of supratentorial intracranial abscess: a review of 200 cases. Br Med J 2:7–9, 1969

7. Greenlee John E: Anatomic considerations in central nervous system infections. pp 725–738. In Mandell GL, Douglas RG, Bennett JE Eds: Principles and Practices of Infectious Diseases. John Wiley and Sons, New York, 1979

8. Wright JLW, Grimaldi PMGB: Otogenic intracranial complications. Laryngol Otol 67:1085–1090, 1973

9. Morgan H, Wood MW: Cerebellar abscesses: a review of 17 cases. Surg Neurol 3:92–96, 1975

10. Kaplan RJ: Neurological complications of infections of the head and neck. Otolaryngol Clin North Am 9:729–738, 1976

11. Yoshikawa TT, Goodman SJ: Brain abscess. West J Med 121:207–219, 1974

12. Outcome of severe damage of the central nervous system. Ciba Foundation Symposium 34. Excerpta Medica, Amsterdam, 1975

13. Underman AE, Overturf GD, Leedom JM: Bacterial Meningitis 1978. February 2:639–650

14. Gotschlich EM: Bacterial meningitis: the beginning of the end. Am J Med 65:719–721, 1978

15. Finegold SM: Central nervous system infection. pp 155–164. In Finegold S Ed: Anaerobic Infections. Academic Press, New York, 1978

16. Zimmerman RA, et al.: Evolution of cerebral abscess: correlation of clinical features with computed tomography. Neurology 27:14–18, 1978

17. New PFJ, Davis KR: The role of CT scanning in diagnosis of infections of the central nervous system. pp 1–33 In Remington J, Swartz M Eds: Current Clinical Topics in Infectious Disease. McGraw-Hill, New York, 1978

18. Heiman HS, Braude A: Anerobic infection of the brain: observation on 18 consecutive cases of brain abscess. Am J Med 35:682–697, 1963

19. Yoshikawa TT: Brain abscess and subdural empyema. pp. 57–62. In Yoshikawa TT, Chow AW, Guze LB Eds: Infectious Diseases: Diagnosis and Management. Houghton Mifflin, Boston, 1980

20. Gantz NM, Gleckman RA. Manual of Clinical Problems in Infectious Disease. pp 158–171. Little, Brown and Co., Boston, 1979

21. Hirschmann JV: Infectious Disease Manual. The Upjohn Co, February 1976

22. Samson DS, Clark K: Current review of brain abscess. Am J Med 54:201–210, 1973

23. Pons VC, Hoff JT: Infections of the CNS. pp 265–275. In Wilson C, Hoff JT Eds: Current Surgical Management of Neurologic Disease. Churchill Livingstone, New York, 1980

24. Heath LK, Goldstun E, Dublin A: Considerations in diagnosing brain abscess with computerized axial tomography. Arch Intern Med 138:628–629, 1978

25. Levenick M: Lecture: Computerized Tomography of the Head. USC School of Medicine. May 1979

26. Sanford JP: Guide to Antimicrobial Therapy 1980. Bristol Laboratories: Division of Bristol-Meyers, 1980

27. Kaufman DM, Miller MH, Slerbigel NH: Subdural empyema. Medicine 54: 485–498, 1975
28. Hitchcock E, Andreadis A: Subdural empyema. J Neurol, Neurosurg, Psychiatry. 27:422–434, 1964
29. Bhandari YS, Sarkari NBS: Subdural empyema: a review of 37 cases. J Neurosurg 32:35–39, 1970
30. Greenlee JE: Subdural empyema. pp 786–788. In Mandell G, Douglas RG Jr, Bennett JE Eds: Principles and Practices of Infectious Diseases. John Wiley and Sons, New York, 1979
31. French LA, Chou SN: Osteomyelitis of the skull and epidural abscess. pp 59–72. In Gurdjian ES Ed; Cranial and Intracranial Suppration. Charles C Thomas, Springfield IL, 1969
32. Swarz MN, Karchner AW: Infections of the central nervous system. pp 309–310. In Belows a, deHaan RM, Dowell VR Jr, et al. Eds: Anaerobic Bacteria: Role in Disease. Charles C Thomas, Springfield IL, 1974
33. LeBeau J, et al.: Surgical treatment of brain abscess and subdural empyema. J Neurosurg 38:198–203, 1973
34. Greenlee JE: Epidural abscess. pp 788–789. In Mandell G, Douglas RG Jr, Bennett JE Eds: Principles and Practices of Infectious Diseases. John Wiley and Sons, New York, 1979
35. Lott T, El Gammal T, DaSilva R, et al.: Evaluation of brain and epidural abscess by computed tomography. Radiology 122:371–376
36. Kaufman DMA, Leeds NE: Computed tomography (CT) in the diagnosis of intracranial abscess. Neurology 27:1069–1075, 1977
37. Sanders WE Jr: Meningitis and encephalitis. pp 351–367. In Cluff Le, Johnson JE Eds: Clinical Concepts of Infectious Diseases 2nd ed. Williams and Wilkins, Baltimore, 1978
38. Wehrle PF: Meningitis. pp 436–453. In Franklin HT Sr, and Wehrle PF Eds: Communicable and Infectious Diseases. CV Mosby, St. Louis, 1976
39. Swartz MN, Dodge PR: Bacterial meningitis. N Engl J Med. 272:725–731, 1965
40. Hoeprich PD: Acute bacterial meningitis. pp 889–901. In Hoeprich PD Ed: Infectious Diseases. Harper and Row, Hagerstown, 1977
41. Wenner HA: Viral meningitis. pp 881–888. In Hoeprich PD Ed: Infecious Diseases. Harper and Row, Hagerstown, 1977
42. Davis JE, Mason CB: Neurological Critical Care. pp 220–226. Van Nostrand Reinhold Co, 1979
43. Yoshikawa TT: Meningitis and encephalitis. pp 45–56. In Yoshikawa TT, Chow AW, Guze LB Eds: Infectious Diseases: Diagnosis and Management. John Wiley and Sons, New York, 1980
44. Overturf GD, Wehrle PF: Bacterial meningitis, which regimen? Drugs 18:65–73, 1979
45. Barrett-Conner E: Tuberculosis meningitis in adults. South Med J 60:1061–1070, 1967
46. Finegold SM: Central nervous system infections. Anaerobic Bacteria in Human Disease, Academic Press, New York, 1977
47. Beaty HN: The central nervous system: meningitis. pp 409–418. In Bennett JV, Brachman PS Eds: Hospital Infections. Little, Brown and Co, Boston, 1979
48. Heerema MS, et al.: Anaerobic bacterial meningitis. Am J Med 67:219–227, 1979
49. Goodman SJ, et al.: Subgaleal abscess, a preventable complication of scalp trauma. West J Med 127:169–172, 1977

50. Conway BL: Neurological trauma. pp 392–398. In Carini and Owens Neurological and Neurosurgical Nursing. CV Mosby, St. Louis, 1978
51. Wright RL: A survey of possible etiologic agents in postoperative craniotomy infections. J Neurosurg 25:125–132, 1966
52. Balch RE: Wound infections complicating neurosurgical procedures. J Neurosurg 26:41–45, 1967
53. Pitts L: Head injury. pp 225–233. In Wilson C, Hoff JT Eds: Current Surgical Management of Neurologic Disease. Churchill Livingstone, New York, 1980
54. Lundberg N: Continuous recording and control of ventricular fluid pressure in neurosurgical practice. Acta Psychiatr Scand 36:1–193 (Suppl 149), 1960
55. Rosner MJ, Becker D: Intracranial pressure monitoring: complications and associated factors. Clin Neurosurg 23:494–519, 1976

9 | Myasthenia Gravis and the Guillain-Barré Syndrome

Mary Blount
Anna Belle Kinney
Nancy Luttrell

This chapter is a general discussion of major considerations for the management of the patient with myasthenia gravis (MG) and the Guillain-Barré syndrome (GBS). It will place emphasis on the similarities between the two disease processes and on the physiologically unstable myasthenic and the GBS patient with ascending paralysis. A complete discussion of these topics and detailed management of these diseases is beyond the scope of this chapter, however, references providing this information have been included. An overview of neuromuscular disorders is presented in a recent article by Donohoe.[3]

This discussion is not limited to critical care nursing because in both these diseases the most crucial period of nursing monitoring is prior to, not after, respiratory failure.

PATHOPHYSIOLOGY

The pathophysiology of MG and GBS are primarily unrelated, however, they have a few common characteristics which are of interest: 1) both are neuromuscular diseases that involve the motor unit (lower motor neuron and the muscle fibers innervated by it); 2) the pathogenesis of each is autoimmune or allergic in nature; and, 3) the development of animal models of each has produced tremendous advances in the understanding of the disease process and its management.

Myasthenia Gravis

MG is almost certainly a systemic autoimmune disease that produces a dysfunction in neuromuscular transmission. Although the most disabling symptom occurs secondary to the disruption of neuromuscular transmission, most treatments are aimed at the underlying autoimmune process.

Autoimmune Process.   The etiology of MG is unknown but there is considerable evidence that the disease is an autoimmune process.[4] This evidence can be summarized as follows: 1) there is a higher-than-expected association of MG with other autoimmune diseases such as systemic lupus erythematosus, rheumatoid arthritis, Hashimoto's thyroiditis, pemphigus and polymyositis; 2) many different autoantibodies have been isolated from the blood of MG patients (e.g., antithymus, antimuscle, antiacetylcholine receptor site); 3) there is a high incidence of thymic abnormalities and favorable response to thymectomy (the thymus is an integral part of the immune system); 4) exacerbations of the disease can be produced by such natural psychological/physiological immunological challenges as surgery, infection, menstruation, pregnancy, and emotional upset and anxiety; and 5) there is often clinical improvement following immunosuppressive therapy. In experimental MG, an autoimmune response is produced in an animal by injecting it with carbachol, α bungarotoxin or α cobratoxin which produces a dysfunction in the acetylcholine receptor sites.

Neuromuscular Transmission.   Nerve impulses transmitted along a lower motor neuron release quanta of acetylcholine (ACh) from vesicles in the terminal axon. The ACh diffuses across the synaptic cleft and interacts with acetylcholine receptor sites in the postsynaptic muscle membrane to produce action potentials which, if of sufficient intensity, result in contraction of muscle fibers. The action of ACh is terminated when it is hydrolyzed by the enzyme acetylcholinesterase (AChE). Past theories of MG pathogenesis have included presynaptic underproduction/storage of ACh and postsynaptic overproduction of AChE. Current investigations have shown that, in fact, there is a simplification of the postsynaptic clefts and a reduction of the number of ACh receptor sites in MG patients. This pathological change results in impaired neuromuscular transmission.

Guillain-Barré Syndrome

The pathogenesis of GBS is less well understood than that of MG. It is, however, considered to be an autoimmune/allergic process that produces segmental demyelination of peripheral nerves.

Autoimmune/Allergic Process.   A significant amount of accumulated evidence supports the theory that GBS is an autoimmune/allergic event.[9] This evidence can be summarized as follows: 1) circulating blood lymphocytes in

GBS patients are sensitized to the basic protein of the peripheral nervous system; 2) the lymphoid blood cells have active DNA synthesis and the mononuclear blood cells are indistinguishable from the mononuclear cells found near the affected nerve roots; 3) GBS is a well documented post-vaccination (particularly post-Swine flu vaccination) complication and is ultrastructurally similar to experimentally induced allergic encephalomyelitis; and 4) many GBS patients report antecedent flu-like infections of the upper respiratory or gastrointestinal tract.

In 1955, an animal model of GBS was developed by injecting rabbits with an emulsion of rabbit sciatic nerve. Approximately 14 days after innoculation, the rabbits developed an allergic neuritis similar to GBS in humans. Coonhound paralysis, a polyradiculitis resembling GBS, may occur naturally after the dog is bitten by a raccoon or experimentally after innoculation of the dog with raccoon saliva.[14]

Peripheral Nervous System. The segmental demyelinating lesions of GBS are confined to the peripheral nervous system and are characterized by localized, scattered destruction of myelin with preservation of the axon, even when the myelin sheath has completely disappeared. The cranial and spinal nerves may be affected anywhere along their lengths—at the roots, the proximal portion, the plexus, or the peripheral nerves. For nerve conduction velocities to be abnormal, the spinal nerves must have demyelination distal to their exit from the vertebral column because, if only the roots are affected, the velocities will be unaltered.

Haymaker and Kernohan described the sequence of events occurring in the nerve roots of patients with GBS[6] (Table 9-1).

CLINICAL PICTURE

Myasthenia Gravis

Myasthenia gravis is a disease characterized by fatigable weakness of voluntary (skeletal) muscles. It has an incidence of approximately 3–6 per 100,000 people, with females being affected much more than males, particularly in the under-40 age group. There do not seem to be racial or socioeconomic factors in disease development.

Any voluntary muscles may be involved, although the most commonly affected are voluntary muscles innervated by cranial nerves. Among the symp-

Table 9-1. Nerve Root Changes with GBS[9]

Days	Changes
1–4	Edema
5–8	Degeneration of myelin sheath with disintegration of the myelin and localized fragmentation of the axis cylinders
9–10	Infiltration with lymphocytes
11–12	Infiltration with phagocytes
13–46	Proliferation of Schwann cells

toms are ptosis, diplopia, dysphagia, dyspnea, and dysphonia. Cranial nerve involvement may exist alone or in association with generalized weakness of one or more extremities.

The weakness in MG increases with muscle use and improves following rest. Most MG patients feel stronger in the morning, but grow increasingly weak as the day progresses. The disease is characterized by exacerbations and remissions. Exacerbations may be the result of stress, infection, or trauma; remissions may be spontaneous or the result of treatment.

Guillain-Barré Syndrome

Guillain-Barré syndrome (also referred to as Landry-Guillain-Barré-Strohl syndrome, infectious polyneuritis, acute idiopathic polyradiculoneuritis) affects persons of all ages and both sexes. Even though many of the patients with GBS report a history of either an upper respiratory, flu-like syndrome or gastroenteric infection approximately 1–3 weeks before the onset of symptoms, the disease does not occur seasonally and may occur without prodrome.

The disease generally progresses rapidly. Clumsiness may be the first symptom the patient notes. The classic case of GBS is an ascending paralysis beginning in the lower extremities which may progress to involve the entire body. The final level of paralysis varies greatly and cannot be predicted. It may only involve the lower extremities or ascend to involve cranial nerves, producing symptoms such as dysphagia, dyspnea, and facial palsies. The dysfunction of GBS is primarily a lower motor neuron type paralysis; the patient may experience paresthesias, however, gross sensation remains intact.

The duration of GBS varies with the level of paralysis. When the paralysis stops progressing, improvement generally begins within 2 weeks. The recovery phase may continue for as long as 6 months to 3 years. Approximately 50% of GBS patients recover totally; of the remaining 50%, 45% are left with a mild residual deficit and only 5% suffer severe disability.

DIAGNOSIS

The clinical history and presentation are the most important elements in the diagnosis of MG and GBS. With MG in particular, a high degree of suspicion is essential for an accurate diagnosis since a significant number of patients are mistakenly diagnosed as neurotic or malingering. GBS patients also may initially be suspected of having psychological disturbances, although less frequently than MG patients. In addition to clinical history and presentation, there are a variety of tests used for diagnosing MG and GBS.

Myasthenia Gravis

If MG is suspected, the Tensilon® test is used first. When Tensilon (edrophonium chloride), a short-acting cholinesterase inhibitor, is injected intravenously, the untreated myasthenic patient will show marked improvement in

30 seconds to 1 minute. This improvement lasts only several minutes, although the length of action varies from patient to patient. A positive Tensilon test strongly supports the diagnosis of MG. On rare occasions, when weakness is limited to the ocular muscles and the Tensilon test is inconclusive, curare may be injected intravenously. Patients with MG are abnormally sensitive to curare. If the patient has MG, the weakness will be exacerbated. However, the danger of acute respiratory failure severely limits the usefulness of this test. If curare is used, an anesthesiologist and emergency respiratory support equipment should be present.

Electromyography (EMG) is often used to confirm the clinical diagnosis of MG. The procedure involves observation of the electrical responses of selected muscle fibers to repetitive stimulation of the motor nerve. Normally, when repetitive supraphysiological stimulation is applied to a motor nerve, the muscle will contract at a constant level. If the affected muscles in a patient with MG are stimulated in a similar way, the muscle fiber contraction quickly shows a progressive decremental response. The single fiber EMG (simultaneous recordings from two individual muscle fibers in the same motor unit) of an MG patient shows a variation in the time response of the two fibers to a single stimulus. This temporal variation is known as *jitter*, which results from unequal neuromuscular transmission time in the two motor endplates.[10]

Other components of the evaluation of the MG patient include investigation of immune status and radiological studies to detect thymic abnormalities.

Guillain-Barré Syndrome

There is no definitive diagnostic test for GBS. Cerebrospinal fluid (CSF) in GBS is normal except for elevated protein levels (50–200 mgm/100 ml). The maximum protein elevation is usually achieved between days 10 and 20. The increased protein level in GBS is the result of elevated levels of immunoglobulins. Electrophoresis and quantitation of immunoglobulins in the CSF show increases in gamma globulins and IgG in a majority of patients.[6]

Nerve conduction studies provide information about the status of myelinated nerves by calculating the velocity with which impulses are transmitted.[12] One stimulating and one recording surface electrode are applied along a peripheral nerve to measure the conduction velocity. In demyelinating peripheral neuropathies such as GBS, conduction velocities are slowed (except when demyelination is limited to the nerve roots).

MANAGEMENT

Management of MG and GBS is similar in many aspects. Management techniques specific to each will be presented first, followed by a discussion of techniques common to the management of both disease processes.

Myasthenia Gravis

Two of the most common methods of treating MG (anticholinesterase drug therapy and thymectomy) are discussed in this section. Two other methods, steroid therapy and plasma exchange, are discussed under Treatment of Autoimmune Process. Other therapies not presented but used experimentally include cytotoxic therapy, thoracic duct drainage, gamma globulins, antilymphocyte and antithymocyte sera and other immunosuppressive agents such as azathioprine (Imuran®).

Anticholinesterase Drug Therapy.   Anticholinesterase drug therapy is not aimed at suppressing the underlying autoimmune process but rather at maximizing neuromuscular transmission. Anticholinesterase drugs inhibit hydrolysis of ACh by AChE. This has the effect of increasing the time during which the available ACh can interact with the diminished number of ACh receptor sites. Thus, by increasing the number of ACh-receptor interactions, neuromuscular transmission is improved.

Anticholinesterase drugs play an important role in both the diagnosis and management of MG. The most commonly used anticholinesterase agents are neostigmine (Prostigmin®), pyridostigmine (Mestinon®) and ambenonium chloride (Mytelase®). These drugs have a duration of approximately 4 hours with peak effect occurring approximately 1 hour after administration. Unfortunately, the correct dosage requirement of any one of these drugs used to treat the MG patient is highly individualized, often difficult to determine, and may change drastically with such factors as stress, surgery, and alterations in therapy modes, commonly occurring during hospitalization.

It is often difficult to distinguish a myasthenic state (anticholinesterase underdosage) from a cholinergic state (anticholinesterase overdosage), as both produce increased weakness. If the weakness produces respiratory failure, the patient is said to be in either a myasthenic (underdosed) or cholinergic (overdosed) crisis. The main clinical features distinguishing the two states are the parasympathetic side effects (e.g., abdominal cramping, increased salivation, diarrhea) often associated with the cholinergic state. The most reliable method for determining whether the patient is underdosed or overdosed is the Tensilon test. Improvement in clinical status (a positive Tensilon test) is indicative of underdosage; exacerbation of weakness and the occurrence or worsening of parasympathetic side effects (a negative Tensilon test) is indicative of overdosage. The parasympathetic side effects produced by the Tensilon (although *not* the weakness), may be controlled by the injection of intravenous atropine. Dosage of the longer acting maintenance anticholinesterase agent is regulated according to Tensilon test results.

Anticholinesterase drugs should always be administered exactly at the scheduled time. Giving the drug too early risks overdosage; a delay in administration may result in the patient being too weak to swallow the drug without first receiving intravenous Tensilon. Strict adherence to a rigid dosage schedule is often unnecessary when the patient is at home, but during hospitalization, control of this variable is essential to accurate interpretation of clinical data.

In addition, it is imperative to know the exact time of anticholinesterase drug administration because Tensilon testing frequently is timed to coincide with the period of least drug effect.

The patient's clinical status should be evaluated and documented at the time of anticholinesterase drug administration—when the patient is weakest. Components of the evaluation include measurement of vital capacity and swallowing ability and a determination of the presence or absence of diplopia and ptosis.[7] Patients whose clinical status fluctuates significantly when taking anticholinesterase drugs must have their activities carefully scheduled to avoid fatigue and to maximize independence in activities of daily living.

Thymectomy. Thymectomy has long been a major therapeutic intervention in the treatment of MG despite the fact that there have been no controlled, prospective studies comparing the results of medical and surgical treatment. On an empirical basis, thymectomy does produce significant benefits for a large number of MG patients. Although there is some controversy over the characteristics of the ideal candidate for surgery, there is evidence that patients meeting the following criteria experience the most benefit: female, under 50 years of age, without thymoma, and without long-standing disease. The benefits of thymectomy are very slow to appear, with improvement frequently not occurring before 1 year and maximum benefit often not achieved for up to 5–7 years.

There is no concensus on the best surgical approach for a thymectomy. Those advocating a median sternotomy (sternal splitting) approach argue that this method provides the best visualization of the chest cavity and thus increases the opportunity for removal of all thymic tissue. Retained thymic tissue may continue to be active and hormone-producing. Those advocating the transcervical approach stress the lowered perioperative mortality rate with this procedure and express doubts that a complete thymectomy is even possible because of the variable location and extension of the thymus.[10]

Thorough preoperative teaching is essential with special emphasis on and practice of postoperative respiratory management techniques (e.g., turning, coughing, and deep breathing exercises accomplished with a spirometer). If the patient is receiving chronic prednisone therapy, supplemental steroids should be administered before, during, and after surgery; adrenal suppression caused by chronic prednisone therapy makes it impossible for the patient to compensate for the stress of surgery without this supplementation.

All patients with MG must be monitored very closely following thymectomy for respiratory status and swallowing ability. This is particularly true of patients receiving anticholinesterase drug therapy. Both the beneficial effects of thymectomy and the adverse effects of surgical stress increase the risk of significant changes in anticholinesterase drug requirements.

Guillain-Barré Syndrome

Much of the care of patients with GBS is the same as for patients with MG. These areas of similarity will be discussed in the following sections. In this section, two problems unique to GBS are presented: autonomic nervous system dysfunction and sensory disturbances.

Autonomic Dysfunction.   Problems with autonomic nervous system function are common in GBS. Those most frequently seen involve incomplete control of blood pressure and heart rate. Both severe hypertension and hypotension have been reported, with many patients exhibiting blood pressure lability and blood pressure fluctuations between the two extremes. In the absence of an arterial line, blood pressure may need to be checked as often as every 5 minutes if problems with control occur. Hypotension is usually managed with a combination of plasma expanders and the Trendelenburg position. Sustained hypertension requires pharmacological management. The most common cardiac abnormalities are tachycardia and arrhythmias. Tachycardia usually responds to a parasympathomimetic agent, such as edrophonium chloride (Tensilon®). Severe and or persistent arrhythmias may require more aggressive therapy. Mechanisms of autonomic dysfunction in GBS are not well understood but have been attributed to involvement of the autonomic nervous system in the disease process and to inappropriate catacholamine release.[11]

Sensory Disturbances.   In their classic 1949 article, Haymaker and Kernohan[6] reported that pain along the distribution of a peripheral nerve occurred in over 50% of their cases, usually as an initial symptom. More than half of their patients also experienced paresthesias, described as numbness or tingling which began in distal extremities and ascended. Pain and tenderness in muscles and joints were also reported. In our experience, many patients only begin to complain of pain during the recovery phase when function is returning.

The etiology of the sensory disturbances is not understood, however, several possible etiologies have been suggested: local re-innervation of wasted muscle, sensory nerve involvement in the demyelinating process, and discomfort secondary to immobility.

In many cases, this pain can be adequately controlled by positioning. If not, a mild analgesic may be necessary. Recently, the use of Dilantin® (phenytoin sodium) or Tegretol® (carbamazepine) has been successful in managing neuralgia of this type.

TREATMENT OF AUTOIMMUNE PROCESS

As described in the section on pathophysiology, both MG and GBS are associated with immune system dysfunction. This is more clearly understood in the case of MG than it is in GBS. Two interventions to control the autoimmune process, steroid therapy and plasma exchange, are of established benefit in the treatment of the disease. Although their efficacy in the management of GBS is less well accepted, these interventions are being used more frequently to treat GBS. There is some reluctance to use steroid therapy and plasma exchange for treating GBS, which is a self-limiting disease, because these interventions are associated with potential side effects, and because, in the case of plasma exchange, the procedure is very expensive.

Steroid Therapy

In an attempt to suppress the autoimmune process, patients with MG are frequently treated with high dose, alternate day, chronic steroid (usually prednisone) therapy or, less commonly, with short courses of adrenocorticotropic hormone. The patient must be monitored closely, usually in an acute care unit, during the initiation of chronic steroid therapy as it is common for an exacerbation to occur anywhere from 1 to 21 days following initiation of treatment. The prednisone dosage is tapered very slowly over months to years as the patient's clinical response permits. The benefits of chronic steroid therapy are well established[13] and a significant number of patients respond by going into remission. Chronic steroid therapy does have many potentially serious side effects and the patient receiving chronic steroid must be monitored closely for their development and appropriate preventive measures must be taken.[1] The development of certain side effects (such as myopathy or severe osteoporosis) require the termination of the therapy.

The use of steroids in the management of GBS remains a subject of some debate. Steroid therapy is a logical consideration because of the suspected autoimmune etiology and the presence of nerve root edema. However, there have been no controlled studies that demonstrate the effectiveness of steroid therapy in decreasing the severity or duration of the illness. Those advocating the use of steroids claim that, when given early in the course of the disease, its progression is slowed and improvement hastened. Those who oppose the use of steroids point out that GBS is a self-limiting disease and that the immunosuppression caused by steroids puts the patient at risk for developing secondary infections.

Plasma Exchange

Plasma exchange is the process of removing whole blood from the patient, centrifuging it into its component parts, removing the plasma, and returning the remainder of the blood (with new plasma or a plasma substitute) to the patient. Plasma exchange has been used to treat a variety of autoimmune disorders, primarily MG. The theoretical basis for plasma exchange is that since autoantibodies circulate in the plasma of patients with MG, if they are removed, the patient should improve.

The procedure is usually done over a course of 2–4 weeks in which exchanges are done every 2–3 days. The patient stays in a reclining position during the entire procedure, which may last several hours. Blood is removed via a 16-gauge $1\frac{1}{4}$ inch angiocath, which is usually inserted into a vein in the antecubital fossa. Following plasma removal, the remaining blood components and plasma replacement are returned to the patient either through a second venous access site or, if venous access is limited, through the same site. A detailed description of the technique of plasma exchange and considerations for patient management is presented in a recent article by Blount et al.[2]

Plasma exchange is not initiated without considerable thought. Not only is it an extremely expensive procedure, it also has potentially serious side effects. The most significant of these are electrolyte imbalances and venous trauma. The most frequent electrolyte imbalances are hypokalemia and hypocalcemia. If problems with venous access occur, it may be necessary to surgically create an arteriovenous fistula, shunt, or graft.

In the treatment of MG, plasma exchange is usually reserved for patients who do not respond satisfactorily to more conventional therapy, those patients having an acute exacerbation of the disease, or those who need to be in optimal condition prior to surgery. Another form of immunosuppression (e.g., chronic steroid therapy, azathioprine therapy) is usually used in conjunction with the plasma exchange. The role of plasma exchange in the management of GBS has not yet been determined. It is being used, however, in several medical centers on an experimental basis with some apparent success.

SYMPTOMATIC CARE

Patients with MG and GBS may require a variety of interventions to control various symptoms. The GBS in particular may require such aids as splints to maintain range of motion, in and out catheterization to compensate for urinary retention, and an aggressive bowel program to prevent constipation. In this section only two areas of physiological function commonly impaired by both MG and GBS will be discussed: ventilation and swallowing.

Ventilation

Respiratory failure is common in both MG exacerbation and GBS. Artificial mechanical ventilation with all its inherent risks is required during this period. However, ventilatory support for these patients is relatively uncomplicated because the failure is due to a problem of neuromuscular control and not the result of pulmonary disease.[8] The most crucial time of nursing management is prior to and not after intubation. It is absolutely essential that the patient with barely compensated respiratory function be monitored extremely closely in order to anticipate incipient respiratory failure. Measurement of vital capacity and/or inspiratory and expiratory pressures give earlier indications of decompensation than does tidal volume. Measurements should be taken with the patient in the sitting position. Very weak patients may need assistance in occluding the nose and obtaining a seal around the mouthpiece of the spirometer.

In both GBS and MG the frequency of respiratory monitoring should be at least every 4 hours. If the MG patient is receiving anticholinesterase medication, measurements should be taken at the time of drug administration when respiratory function is presumably at its lowest. The frequency of monitoring should be increased if the patient's physical condition appears to be deteriorating. Care must be taken not to inadvertently produce respiratory failure by taxing the respiratory muscles with overzealous monitoring. "Over-monitoring" of the GBS patient is of less concern as the progression of the paralysis is largely independent of fatigue.

Once adequate respiratory function has returned, weaning the MG or GBS patient from mechanical ventilatory support is usually not difficult. When problems do occur, they are generally the result of either premature weaning or patient anxiety.

Swallowing

Dysphagia, like dyspnea, is a problem common to both MG and GBS. Inability to swallow is usually managed with a nasogastric tube. Also, as in the case of respiratory failure, the most critical period is not following but prior to therapeutic intervention. Careful monitoring is essential to identify decompensation of swallowing ability before aspiration occurs, as aspiration alone can precipitate respiratory failure.

Unfortunately it is not uncommon for swallowing to be tested by having the patient attempt to swallow substances of various consistencies. This method entails the risk of aspiration if swallowing ability is overestimated. It is much safer to rely on a subjective method of evaluation wherein the patient swallows nothing but saliva and then estimates his or her swallowing ability (Table 9-2).

The timing and frequency of monitoring is determined according to the same guidelines discussed in the section on ventilation. If there is any question concerning the adequacy of the patient's swallowing, suctioning equipment should be installed at the bedside. If an MG patient's swallowing ability fluctuates with anticholinesterase administration, meals may have to be ordered to coincide with peak drug effect.

SUPPORTIVE CARE

The acute phases of both MG and GBS are temporary in nature although intensive nursing care may be required for days, weeks, and on rare occasions, months. It is the responsibility of the staff to ensure that the patient suffers no preventable complications from immobility during the critical period of illness that will impede the subsequent rehabilitation process. Interventions to counteract the effects of immobility have been extensively documented. The fact is that in the modern hospital the patient with MG or GBS is at far greater risk of complications (or death) from the effects of immobility than from the effects of the primary disease. With rare exception, the development of such complications as pressure sores, contractures, bacterial and/or aspiration pneumonia, and urinary tract infections are inversely related to the quality of nursing care delivered.

Table 9-2. Scale for Estimating Swallowing Ability[2]

0 = Unable to swallow anything
1 = Able to swallow saliva only
2 = Able to swallow liquids
3 = Able to swallow pureed foods
4 = Able to swallow a soft diet
5 = Able to swallow a regular diet

The second major problem area in which supportive nursing care is required is anxiety. The patient whose breathing and swallowing abilities are threatened by MG or GBS has intact mental and sensory functions and is bedridden, essentially quadraplegic, and in fear of imminent death. He or she must constantly be reassured that the situation is well under control and that the severe weakness is temporary. The nursing staff should keep the patient well informed of progress being made, explain the rationale for all treatments, and provide advance warning of any interventions. Not only is this constant reassurance humane, but in cases of barely compensated neuromuscular dyspnea and dysphagia, severe anxiety may produce respiratory and swallowing decompensation and failure.

REFERENCES

1. Blount M, Kinney AB: Chronic steroid therapy. Am J Nurs 74:1626–1631, 1974.
2. Blount M, Kinney AB, Stone M: Plasma exchange in the management of myasthenia gravis. Nurs Clin North Am 14:173–190, 1979.
3. Donohoe KM: An overview of neuromuscular disease. Nurs Clin North Am 14:95–106, 1979.
4. Drachman DB: Myasthenia gravis. I. N Engl J Med 298:136–142, 1978.
5. Drachman DB: Myasthenia Gravis. II. N Engl J Med 298:186–193, 1978.
6. Haymaker W, Kernohan JW: The Landry-Guillain Barré syndrome: a clinicopathologic report of fifty fatal cases and a critique of the literature. Medicine 28:59–141, 1949.
7. Kinney AB, Blount M: Systems approach to myasthenia gravis. Nurs Clin North Am 6:435–453, 1971.
8. Mayer R, Koski CL: Treatment of acute respiratory muscle failure. In Saleman M, Ed.: Neurologic Emergencies. Raven Press, New York, 1980.
9. Morariu MA: Major Neurological Syndromes. Charles C. Thomas: pp. 3–19, Springfield, Illinois, 1979.
10. Patten BM: Myasthenia gravis: review of diagnosis and management. Muscle and Nerve 1:190–205, 1978.
11. Polk BV: Cardiopulmonary complications of Guillain-Barré syndrome. Heart Lung 5:967–969, 1976.
12. Ross AJ et al: Neuromuscular diagnostic procedures. Nurs Clin North Am 14:107–121, 1979.
13. Sanders DB, et al: High dose prednisone in the treatment of myasthenia gravis. In Dau PC Ed: Plasmapheresis and the Immunobiology of Myasthenia gravis. Houghton-Mifflin, Boston, 1979.
14. Holmes DF et al: Experimental coonhound paralysis: animal model of Guillain-Barré syndrome. Neurology 29:1186–1187, 1979.

Index

Page numbers followed by f represent figures; page numbers followed by t represent tables.